POLLUTANTS
AND ANIMALS

POLLUTANTS AND ANIMALS

A Factual Perspective

F. Moriarty
Ph.D.

Monks Wood Experimental Station,
Institute of Terrestrial Ecology

London   George Allen & Unwin Ltd
Ruskin House   Museum Street

Printed in Great Britain by Page Bros (Norwich) Ltd,
Mile Cross Lane, Norwich

To Leila

Preface

Pollution affects us all, many of the problems are intrinsically interesting, and during the last decade it has become possible to impose some order on the welter of facts that has accumulated. Nevertheless much of the material available to people who are not closely involved is trivial or misleading. I hope this book will enable readers to understand the scientific problems of pollution in greater depth, and prompt them to ask the important questions, because public pressure is one of the most effective means of ensuring that pollution problems are tackled effectively. It is probably true to say that, but for Rachel Carson's 'Silent Spring', my job for one would never have been created.

The writing of this book has been helped greatly by the catalytic effect of my colleagues in the Toxic Chemicals and Wildlife Section at Monks Wood. They have helped to stimulate my ideas, and many of the examples quoted come from their work. I thank, first of all, Dr N. W. Moore, founder member and head of the section, whose immense experience has been an invaluable touchstone. I would also like in particular to thank Dr A. S. Cooke, Dr B. N. K. Davis, Dr J. P. Dempster—now head of the section for invertebrate population ecology—Mr M. C. French, Dr D. J. Jefferies, Mr C. Newbold and Mr J. L. F. Parslow. I must also thank two former colleagues, Mr I. Prestt and Dr D. A. Ratcliffe, now with the new Nature Conservancy Council. Finally I must record my debt to Professor K. Mellanby, who so contrived Monks Wood that it has been a most stimulating and fulfilling place in which to work.

I would also like to thank Dr P. S. Hewlett and Mr M. Owens for their comments on some parts of the book.

My wife has provided constant advice and help. To her I am most grateful.

F. MORIARTY

Monks Wood Experimental Station

Acknowledgements

I am indebted to the following individuals and organisations for permission to reproduce some of the figures and tables in this book: the editors of the *Annals of Applied Biology* for permission to reproduce Fig. 6–1 and the data on p. 87; the editors of *Bird Study* for the data on p. 46; the publishers of the *Entomologists Gazette* for Fig. 6–2; the editor of *Environmental Pollution* for Fig. 2–3; the editors of the *Journal of Applied Ecology* for Fig. 3–1, and for the data on pp. 43 and 95; the editor of *Nature* for Fig. 5–4, Tables 4–1 and 4–2 and for the data on p. 84; the editor of the *Science of the Total Environment* for Fig. 5–2 and Tables 5–1, 5–2 and 5–4; the publishers of *Toxicology and Applied Pharmacology* for Fig. 7–2; and the Controller of Her Majesty's Stationery Office for the data on p. 129.

Contents

Figures

Tables

I

Introduction

Pollution of our environment has occurred for centuries, but it has only become a significant problem within the last few decades. Our species' impact on the environment is no longer minuscule: both our numbers and our technology have increased greatly. We cannot now, for example, pour our untreated sewage direct into rivers without gross effects on the wildlife there, because our sewage has increased both in amount and sorts.

I mean by the term pollutant a substance that occurs in the environment as a result of man's activities, and which has a deleterious effect on living organisms. Both of these criteria, of man's activities and of damage, are important. There are many naturally occurring substances that have deleterious effects on at least some species—even too much chalk or lime in the soil will inhibit the development of many plant species. On the other hand, many of the chemicals which we release into the environment do not appear to have any adverse effects, at least within very wide limits.

This definition of pollutants is somewhat restricted, and often the term is used to include noise and other forms of energy. Personally I find this wider use unsatisfactory. The term then includes disparate phenomena, and it almost becomes synonymous with 'everything I don't like'. One definition includes 'substances or energy patterns' that 'offend' one. This means that one man's pollutant, such as cigarette smoke, may be another man's meat. There are perfectly valid and well-established words, such as nuisance, to describe these other activities.

Whether or not a substance is a pollutant depends not only on what it is, but also on where it is. Nitrates and phosphates are beneficial as artificial fertilisers when applied to arable crops in suitable quantities. They are essential nutrients too for plant life in rivers. But if so much enters the river from the soil and sewage that algal blooms occur, then these plant nutrients have become pollutants.

It has in fact come as a shock to many people when they first realise that man's activities can, if uncontrolled, have widespread unintended effects on living organisms. The main biological problem is not one of local gross contamination, such as that caused by waste tips from mineral extraction: some of the biological effects of this can clearly be seen, and the main difficulties are administrative. Nor is it one of acute toxicity such as may happen after an accident. One or two barrels of the insecticide endosulfan were accidentally dropped into the Rhine a few years ago. All our newspapers had articles about it because of the enormous number of dead fish that were then seen floating downstream. The main problem is far more difficult to tackle. Do pollutants have more subtle, less obvious, sublethal deleterious effects on life? Insecticides provided the first examples that aroused widespread public concern, and even now most of our framework of ideas relates to these compounds, although one hopes that these ideas are also applicable to other pollutants too.

We must consider two attitudes of mind before we can attempt a rational analysis of this question. The term 'chemical' sometimes has emotional overtones, which do not help logical discussion. This is well illustrated by the preference some people have for farmyard manure as opposed to artificial fertilisers. The one is 'natural', the other is 'chemical'. In fact, both have virtues and defects, both are useful, both can be misused. More to the point, both consist entirely of chemicals: there is no magic in 'muck'. All substances consist entirely of elements and their compounds. Nor is there any difference between naturally occurring compounds and those that are made in the laboratory or factory. Pure ethyl alcohol synthesised from ethylene and sulphuric acid will produce exactly the same results as pure ethyl alcohol extracted from sugars after natural fermentation by yeast.

Secondly, many pollutants are definitely poisons. That is, small amounts have toxic effects. This fact sometimes induces an attitude akin to a neurosis—a fear that any amount of such substances, no matter how small, must be harmful. Fairly recently there was a scare that tinned tuna sold in Great Britain had been polluted with mercury. This scare started in the USA, where the Food and Drug Administration had established a maximum permissible level of 0.5 ppm (parts per million) of mercury in edible fish. Analysis of some tins of tuna had revealed higher levels, and there was the presumption that this tuna had been polluted with mercury as a result of man's activities. Further work showed that such amounts were in fact of natural origin. Museum specimens of tuna caught between 1878 and 1909 had concentrations similar to those in tuna caught recently.

Conversely it must be admitted that there are some who seem unable, or unwilling, to admit the possibility that pollutants have effects, at least on wildlife. They demand far more rigorous proof than is usual in scientific disputes, and tend to ignore or falsify the available facts. To be always right is impossible, but one has an obligation to try to be reasonable.

It is also worth considering for a moment whether it matters anyway if wildlife is affected. And here I am using a wide definition of wildlife, to indicate all undomesticated and uncultivated species of the plant and animal kingdoms. At a personal level, the answer will depend on the individual. Wildlife is, at least consciously, of little or no significance for many people, but there is in Great Britain a strong traditional interest in natural history, which is now flourishing. We have even had for nearly a quarter of a century a government research organisation, the Nature Conservancy[1], whose sole concern is conservation. Wildlife is obviously important for various sports—fishing, shooting, fox-hunting and so on. But the possible elimination of species has other consequences too. Plant breeders for example are already becoming concerned at the loss of plant species that are potentially valuable sources of genetic characters of use in developing new cultivated varieties. I must add that the danger here comes at present from destruction of habitat rather than from pollution.

We could, with proper exploitation, obtain an enormous amount of food from the sea. Pollution could quite conceivably reduce this potential source of food. To take one simple example, many sea fish breed in coastal and estuarine waters, where many pollutants occur in relatively high concentration. Such species could then easily be affected in their spawning grounds. I am not trying to paint a picture of woe and disaster, but I do want to make three points. It is conceivable that pollution could destroy many animal and plant populations: it has already done so. It is undesirable that this should occur unwittingly, because wildlife is, for many people, one of the pleasures of life, and because wildlife is also important scientifically and economically. Our technological revolution has reached the stage where natural resources can no longer be ever-bountiful, unless we manage the environment in a suitable manner: we need to make conscious decisions about how we want to manage our environment.

Questions about the effects of pollutants on living organisms fall into four categories: how much pollutant is present, what effects does it have, what do we want to do about it, and how can we do it? The first two types of question require scientific and technological knowledge for their answers. We already have much of the necessary information for control, although there are large and important gaps. We then need an economic assessment of all the costs of the available

[1] A new Nature Conservancy Council was established on 1st November, 1973.

B

options. But the answers to some of the questions of cost transcend economics, and require value judgements. What, for example, is the value of our wildlife? Some components can be measured in terms of money, but some, such as the enjoyment to be obtained from bird-watching or angling, cannot. A White Paper issued by the British government said aptly 'Government can and must give a lead. But success will also depend on an increasingly informed and active public opinion'. Because many important factual questions cannot yet be answered with certainty, our value judgements must rest on the uncertain base of a balance of probabilities. It is most important then that the nature of these uncertainties be understood, if we are to have an effective public debate and agreement about the control of pollution. Finally we need to devise an effective legal and administrative framework to supervise the control.

I shall devote myself in this book to the first two problems: of how we can measure amounts and effects of a pollutant. The difficulties are not entirely peculiar to pollution. The pharmaceutical industry is asking similar questions. It has been painfully obvious since the thalidomide tragedy that we cannot always predict with certainty all of the effects that a drug may have. So some of their experience is relevant to our problems. For simplicity however, I shall use one small group of compounds, the organochlorine insecticides, for many of my illustrations. They have been one of the star turns so far in public discussion about pollution, and partly because of this we know, relatively, quite a lot about them.

2

Insecticides

DDT is probably the first compound that most people will think of when they hear the word insecticide. It has many remarkable properties, has been much studied, and well repays detailed consideration—it illustrates ideas that help us to understand, and perhaps to solve, the problems posed by pollution in general.

DDT does not occur naturally, and its synthesis was first recorded by O. Zeidler, a German research chemist, in 1874. This compound then received little further attention until about the beginning of the Second World War, when P. Müller, working for the Geigy Company in Switzerland, discovered that it has remarkable insecticidal properties. DDT was not the first insecticide, but its predecessors were of very limited effectiveness. They consisted principally of various inorganic compounds, especially metallic compounds such as lead arsenate, organic compounds such as nicotine and pyrethrins that were extracted from plants, and a few other groups of organic compounds.

By contrast, DDT combined three noteworthy features: it had unprecedented persistence, it was toxic to a very wide range of insect pests, and under normal conditions of use it had low mammalian toxicity. In consequence it was at one time regarded as a paragon of all the virtues. And there is no doubt that the virtues are considerable. It has saved probably millions of lives, by control of insect vectors of diseases and of crop pests. However, subsequent experience has shown that it produces problems too.

We will examine some of these problems in later chapters, but I would like first to consider how DDT acts. Like all poisons, it is toxic in small amounts, but even so, it is important to realise that different molecules of DDT within the body follow different pathways. DDT may enter an animal either through the external body surface, or, if present in the food, from the gut wall. Either way, it is then carried round the body by the blood or circulatory system. In general terms there are then four possible pathways for each molecule of DDT:

Some DDT may be converted into other compounds. In technical terms, some molecules are metabolised. There are several metabolic pathways for DDT, and one of the most commonly found metabolites is DDE. This conversion can be symbolised:

The technical details of this conversion need not concern lay readers. The important point to grasp is that one possible fate for molecules of DDT, or of any other toxic compound, within the body is that they can be metabolised (converted) to other compounds. These metabolites are frequently less toxic to the organism than the parent compound, but, as we shall see later, they are sometimes more toxic.

The details are not fully known of all DDT's metabolic pathways. For example, DDD is another residue, similar in structure to DDT, that is also commonly found in wildlife specimens:

p,p'- DDD

It is an insecticide in its own right, but it is not used very much in Great Britain. It can also be formed from DDT by various micro-organisms in anaerobic conditions. There is some argument about its source in vertebrates. Some workers consider it to be a normal metabolite, produced by live animals from DDT. However, it has been shown that DDD is rapidly formed after death by micro-organisms present in the tissues, and there is little good evidence to prove that it is a normal metabolite of DDT in live vertebrates.

The importance of different metabolic pathways varies from species to species, and, with a few notable exceptions, very little attention has been paid so far to the possible biological effects of the metabo-lites of pollutants in general. In part this is because it is often technically difficult to discover what metabolites are formed, in part because of an implicit assumption that once the original pollutant has been metabolised it has also been detoxified. Even for DDT, which is most commonly found in wildlife specimens as its metabolite DDE, we know relatively little about the effects of DDE. It is usually far less lethal than DDT, but there is evidence to show that it can have sublethal effects, at least in birds.

The second possibility, both for DDT and its metabolites, is that they are excreted from the body. Obviously this is, for the organism, the most satisfactory result. There is then no possibility of future damage. Metabolism is often an essential preliminary to excretion, because metabolites are often more easily excreted than the original molecules. DDE is in fact not such a metabolite. It appears to persist longer within organisms than does DDT.

Molecules of DDT can be found in all parts of an organism, although some tissues, especially tissues with a high fat content, contain higher concentrations than others. In most of these tissues the DDT may be said to be stored, because, so far as we know, it has little or no effect on the organism.

Finally we come to the important, but little used, idea of the site of action. Living organisms stay alive by maintaining many internal processes and states at very constant levels. For example, birds and mammals maintain remarkably constant body temperatures, with elaborate control systems to prevent any marked deviation from the norm. Different species have different normal body temperatures, but most regulate their temperature within close limits; the animal will die if the temperature becomes either too high or too low. Similarly there are many other physiological activities that must continue within controlled limits if the animal is to stay alive. Now pollutants, other poisons and drugs can often be shown, by detailed examination, to produce many deviations from these normal limits, and if the dose is large enough, the deviations are so great that the animal dies. However, these changes are usually secondary, and stem from one single primary, biochemical, lesion which can be defined as the initial biochemical change that occurs within tissue cells. It is often very difficult to discover the details of this biochemical lesion, but there is some information for DDT.

The first obvious symptom of poisoning is usually some form of hyperactivity. Some insects convulse to such an extent that they may cast off one or more of their legs, which still continue to twitch spasmodically. This hyperactivity suggests that DDT interferes with the nervous system in some way.

We have just seen that animals have to regulate many bodily functions if they are to stay alive. The nervous system is one of the principal means of achieving this control, and can be considered as a very complex control system built up from two basic units—axons and synapses. The axons, along which nerve impulses travel, are long extensions of the nerve cells. The ends of these axons lie in close proximity to the ends of axons from other nerve cells, although they do not actually meet, and so form a network which extends throughout the organism. These gaps between axons are called synapses. This network co-ordinates the impulses received from sensory cells and then transmits impulses to the appropriate muscles and glands. The organism can therefore respond effectively to its environment. Thus two different processes control the transfer of information within the nervous system: conduction of impulses along the axons, and conduction of impulses across the synapses.

DDT interferes with the nervous system by increasing the number of impulses that pass along an axon in response to a stimulus. This can obviously explain, in general terms, why animals become hyperactive, although we do not yet know in complete detail how DDT affects the conduction of impulses. There are several theories to choose from, but we can say that DDT produces its primary lesion in the nerve axons. Eventually, if the exposure is large enough, the organism becomes unco-ordinated in its behaviour, then prostrate, and finally dies. The primary lesion is in the nervous system, but death only ensues after many other secondary changes have occurred. The details of all these changes are not known precisely, but it is probably unrealistic to think in terms of a single final effect. Rather, death occurs because the primary lesion disrupts many of the normal control mechanisms so much that the organism can no longer function in a co-ordinated way.

In brief, DDT, or any other pollutant, will kill an organism if sufficient molecules avoid metabolism, storage and excretion, and so reach the site of action, where they initiate a chain of events which upsets the normal physiological balance that is a prerequisite for life. These four pathways should not be considered as completely exclusive of each other: the distribution of DDT within the body is dynamic, not static. For example, a molecule of DDT stored in the tissues may later be metabolised, excreted or transferred to the site of action. Explanations for differences in toxicity to different species must be sought in terms of differences in these four pathways. Other things being equal, a species that can excrete a pollutant rapidly is likely to withstand a higher dose than a species that cannot excrete that pollutant.

Some DDT escapes into rivers with factory effluent from industrial processes such as the moth-proofing of wool. This can also happen of course in factories that manufacture DDT. Moreover, DDT used for agriculture, public health and forestry is released deliberately into the environment. So it should be no surprise that residues of DDT can be found in specimens of wildlife. However, sublethal exposures, if high enough, can produce deleterious effects, so it has been a matter of some concern that DDT, or more commonly its metabolite DDE, has been found in wildlife specimens in most parts of the world, including the Antarctic, often far from any known sources of DDT. The amounts found are often minute, but they do suggest that DDT must be rather persistent, with the corollary that perhaps, if we continue to use DDT at the same or higher rates as we have during the last decade, then amounts in the physical environment and in wildlife may increase.

One must first distinguish clearly between persistence within organisms and persistence in the physical environment. Many chemical processes occur far more quickly within organisms than they do in the environment, in part because they are catalysed by specific proteins known as enzymes. This explains why many animals can lose half of their DDT within a few weeks, largely by metabolism, whereas it is far more persistent in the physical environment.

The molecule of DDT is very stable and resistant to chemical change in the soil, so that only a minor percentage is transformed to other compounds. All the same it is perhaps surprising to find that about half of the DDT applied to arable soil is still present some three years later. This is an average figure for temperate parts of the world, and under some conditions half of the DDT may still be present after ten or more years. This great persistence indicates that DDT is not easily leached from the soil in water, and evaporates into the air very slowly. In fact DDT is so insoluble in water, and has such a low vapour pressure, that both values are very difficult to measure exactly. The best estimate of solubility suggests that water dissolves slightly more than one part of DDT in 10^9 (one thousand million) parts of water. However, poor solubility is not the only reason for the slow leaching of DDT from soil—much of it is often strongly adsorbed onto the surfaces of soil particles. It can be very difficult to wash DDT down a column of soil by passing water through.

It was commonly thought at one time that most of the DDT that disappeared from agricultural soils had been transferred to the rivers with the excess rainwater, either in solution or attached to soil particles. This now seems an unlikely explanation; it has been estimated that the annual rainfall in the USA would remove, in this manner, annually, about 0.1 % of the annual production of DDT in the USA. This is far too low a figure to account for much of the DDT that disappears from soils. This calculation depends on estimates of the average concentration of DDT in river water, and of the amount of water flowing into the seas from the rivers. The conclusion is probably sound, but there is one uncertainty, about the role of sediments on the river bed. For example, it was found in England that DDT could only be detected in river water from Essex and Kent when the local orchards had been heavily sprayed with DDT. Concentrations were rarely much more than one hundred parts or so of DDT per 10^{12} (million million) parts of water. But mud from the bed of one of these rivers, the Chelmer, was later found to contain 10,000–40,000 parts of DDT per 10^{12}. Clearly the mud is an important site for holding DDT, but we do not know how long it has taken for these residues to accumulate in the mud, nor do we know how long the DDT molecules remain in one spot on the river bed.

It has been realised for a long time that when DDT is sprayed onto a crop much of the insecticide never reaches the soil or plant surface at all, but is lost as vapour in the air straight away. As much as 50 % is commonly said never to reach the ground. More DDT volatilises into the air again soon after application. Recent work suggests that this process of volatilisation continues, more slowly, even with DDT that is incorporated into the soil. Laboratory experiments and theoretical calculations suggest that between a few tenths of a pound and one to two pounds of DDT per acre could be lost annually by volatilisation. Little allowance has been made in these calculations however for the effects of soil moisture. Particles of dry soil often retain DDT tenaciously, so that its rate of evaporation will be reduced. Water molecules tend to displace DDT molecules. Moreover, as water evaporates from the soil surface more water will move up to the surface from deeper layers. More DDT will consequently come to the surface in solution. DDT can only diffuse back, down the concentration gradient, into the soil again at a negligible rate, so that its concentration at the surface, which affects evaporation rate, could be much greater than in deeper layers of soil.

The consensus of opinion appears then to favour the idea that most of the DDT in arable soil disappears as vapour into the air, although there is scope for much argument about the details. It is important to grasp the point that disappearance of DDT from the soil does not necessarily mean that it has disappeared altogether. Much, or most, of it has simply moved to another place. If we expect to continue using DDT in considerable amounts indefinitely, then we need to comprehend the total pattern of distribution and loss for DDT, so that we can try to predict any problems that may arise before they occur.

The first obvious question is, how much DDT is being made? It might seem a simple matter to obtain firm data on the total production of DDT, and to make intelligent guesses for the next few years ahead. Manufacturers in the USA do make annual returns for their production of DDT (Fig. 2-1), and there was a fairly steady increase

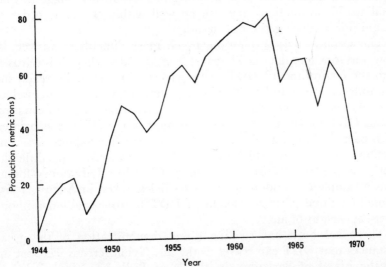

Fig. 2-1. Figures from the annual reports of the 'United States Tariff Commission. United States Production and Sales.' Production figures before 1944 and after 1970 are included with those for other synthetic insecticides

in the amount produced until the peak was reached in 1963, when more than 80,000 metric tons were produced. Production does not necessarily imply that the DDT was actually used that year, nor does it tell us what the DDT was eventually used for—possibly 70% of the United States' production was exported—but nonetheless it is a useful figure to have. Production declined after 1963, and by 1970 had reached such a low level that subsequent figures for DDT production were combined with those for other minor insecticides.

Unfortunately we do not have comparable figures for other countries, where firms are sometimes very reluctant to give production figures for insecticides. The resistance is based principally on the belief that it is against a firm's interests to release such figures. This belief is often held sincerely, although it is difficult to defend rationally, particularly for firms that talk of their social responsibilities. Of course, to be fair, it is not only private enterprises that are reluctant to give information—even the Civil Service is not entirely immune from unnecessary secrecy.

It has been estimated that, during the 1960s, the USA produced about half of the world's total amount of DDT. The situation is different for this decade. Much less DDT is now used in the USA and western Europe because of concern about its great persistence, but much is still used in tropical and subtropical parts of the world for agriculture and public health. Informed guesswork suggests that total world production may still be well within the same order of magnitude as during the last decade.

The second obvious question, much more difficult to answer, is, how and to where does DDT travel from the sites where it is released into the environment? DDT in the rivers will eventually reach the sea, unless retained indefinitely in the sediments, which are themselves of course not entirely static. There are several pieces of information about DDT in the air. It seems that most of the DDT is associated with particles, so that relatively little occurs as free vapour. Concentrations are very low, which makes definitive measurements difficult. For example, the British Government Chemist's Laboratory found that a sample of London air, with particles, taken in August, 1965, contained three parts by weight of DDT to 10^{12} (million million) parts by weight of air.

There has been one striking direct demonstration of the great distances that DDT can travel in the air. Nylon screens were set up on the island of Barbados, in the West Indies, to trap air-borne particles. It was possible to show that most of the trapped particles must have been blown, by the equatorial easterlies, from Europe and Africa, which are more than 6,000 Km away. Analysis showed that these particles carried various insecticides, the principal component being DDT.

DDT can be removed from the air either by falling rain or by dry deposition of particles. There are a few data from various parts of the world, of the amounts of DDT in air, rainwater, and associated with particles, but it is not easy to gain an overall picture of the amounts present, or to estimate rates of transfer. It is possible to argue that the figures for volatilisation of DDT into the air and final deposition into the sea do not account for all of the DDT that enters the atmosphere. This argument is tentative, but throws up one important assumption, that molecules of DDT are stable whilst in the atmosphere. Reports of recent work by K. W. Moilanen and D. G. Crosby in the usa show that when DDT vapour is irradiated with ultraviolet light, of similar wavelength to that found in the atmosphere, some of the DDT is converted to DDE, which is then finally transformed into various chlorinated biphenyls (PCBs):

Biphenyl

We shall discuss PCBs later in this chapter. It is sufficient for the moment to note that both DDE and PCBs do occur in the environment, but we do not know how much is formed by this conversion. It is at present an open question whether this reaction is an important one in the atmosphere.

Eventually much of the DDT that has been released into the environment must end up in the oceans, transported by either rivers or wind. So far as I know, DDT has not yet been detected in ocean water. Presumably some DDT is present, but it is below the present limits of detection. DDT is very poorly soluble in water, and, correlated with this property, it is highly soluble in fats. Fatty tissues in animals invariably have much higher concentrations of DDT than do other tissues, and aquatic animals in general take up DDT very rapidly from the water, and may contain concentrations of DDT several thousand times as large as that in the ambient water. Much of the DDT in the ocean is probably associated with particles or occurs in the very thin fatty layer that often occurs naturally on the surface. Eventually it may penetrate with organic sediments through the surface waters of the ocean and be deposited at the bottom of the abyss.

It should be apparent that much of the last section has been speculative, because we lack firm evidence, and it has certainly not been very quantitative. Ideally we would like to know for each component, or 'sink', of the environment, how much DDT occurs within that component, and, equally important, how rapidly DDT enters and leaves that component. We could then try to make a budget, for any given input of DDT to the environment, of its future distribution and fate.

I have ignored any influence that living organisms might have on the distribution of DDT. G. M. Woodwell *et al* have calculated that the relative masses of living organisms and of their environment are such that animals and plants contain altogether about as much DDT as was produced in three or four days during the mid-1960s. So, although organisms may contain relatively very high concentrations of DDT, they do not appear to have significant large-scale effects on the distribution of DDT.

There is one important detail to be considered about DDT before we consider some other insecticides. So far I have referred to DDT as though it were a single pure compound. In practice, the technical grade DDT that is manufactured for commercial use contains about 30% impurities. One of these is another isomer of DDT. Isomers are molecules made up of the same atoms, but with different dispositions of the atoms within the molecule. This second isomer is called *ortho-para* (or *op'*) DDT, to distinguish it from the main constituent, *para-para* (or *pp'*) DDT, and they differ in the position of one chlorine atom:

p.p'– DDT   *o,p'*– DDT

op'-DDT is also insecticidal, but it is less toxic than the *pp'* isomer. It is this technical grade DDT which is then used in various formulations for specific applications. The formulation is exceedingly important, and can alter the effective toxicity greatly. For example, a formulation for use on plants will ensure that as much of the spray as possible adheres to, and remains on, the plant surface.

I have considered DDT in some detail, because it illustrates some important ideas. It was one of the first of the synthetic insecticides, which we will now review briefly. There are two main groups of these insecticides, organochlorine and organophosphorus. They are so called because they are organic compounds, i.e. the molecule is based on a skeleton of carbon atoms. The organochlorine insecticides also contain chlorine atoms, whilst the organophosphorus insecticides have a phosphorus atom in the centre of the molecule.

There are three main types of organochlorine insecticides, one of which includes DDT and similar compounds such as DDD (also called TDE). The second type consists solely of HCH (hexachlorocyclohexane):

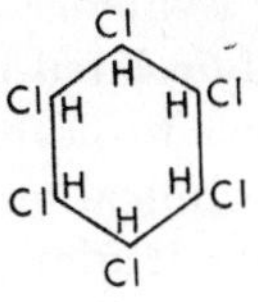

HCH

Unfortunately it is usually misnamed, and called BHC (short for benzene hexachloride), which is in fact a different compound without hydrogen atoms:

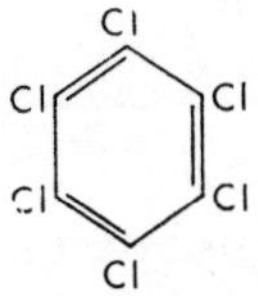

Benzene hexachloride

Technical HCH contains five isomers, of which γ-HCH has by far the highest insecticidal activity. Only 8–15 % of this isomer occurs in technical HCH, so the pure isomer (lindane) is often used. It is one of the most soluble of the organochlorine insecticides, but a saturated solution in water still only contains about ten parts per million of lindane. It is also relatively volatile, so disappears from soils fairly quickly, and it is metabolised rapidly by many organisms. Like DDT, it came into use during the Second World War. The third group, the cyclodienes, were developed after the war. I shall refer most frequently to dieldrin, which, strictly, indicates the technical product, but is often taken to be synonymous with the active principle, HEOD:

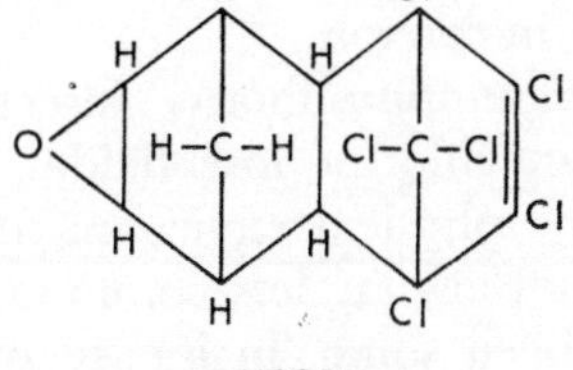

HEOD

Other compounds of this type include aldrin, endrin and heptachlor.

As a group, the organochlorine insecticides are almost insoluble in water, soluble in fats, chemically very stable, and persistent in the physical environment. So far as our knowledge extends, all appear to produce their primary lesion in the nerve axon, although the details differ between insecticides. Evidence is appearing which suggests that for dieldrin it is a closely related metabolite, not dieldrin itself, which is toxic. We know next to nothing about many of the other compounds present in the technical grade products.

The organophosphorus insecticides differ in several ways. There are many types, and I shall only illustrate two examples:

$$CH_3O \atop CH_3O \Big\rangle P-SCHCOOC_2H_5 \atop CH_2COOC_2H_5$$

Malathion

$$CH_3O \atop CH_3O \Big\rangle P-O-CHCl_2$$

Dichlorvos

The early organophosphorus insecticides, such as parathion, had a high acute toxicity for man, and they caused many deaths in various parts of the world. They have been replaced to a large extent by less hazardous compounds. Malathion is a good example. It is effective against many insect pests, but has a low mammalian toxicity. This difference depends on differences in metabolism. Malathion is not toxic until it is converted to malaoxon, when the central phosphorus atom exchanges the sulphur atom for an oxygen atom:

$$\Big\rangle \overset{S}{\underset{P-}{\|}} \longrightarrow \Big\rangle \overset{O}{\underset{P-}{\|}}$$

Malathion   Malaoxon

Both mammals and insects can convert malathion to malaoxon, but in general mammals can degrade both malathion and malaoxon more rapidly than can insects, so that they are far less likely to acquire toxic levels of malaoxon.

Generally these organophosphorus insecticides are far more reactive than the organochlorine insecticides, and are not nearly so persistent, either in the physical environment or within organisms. Because of this, residues are far less common in wildlife specimens, although there have been some 'incidents' of wildlife poisoned by organophosphorus insecticides. Their mode of action is rather different too.

The symptoms of poisoning follow the same general pattern as for organochlorine insecticides, but the primary lesion occurs at the synapse, not in the axon. Impulses are transmitted between axons, across the synapses, by release of a transmitter substance from the end of one axon, some of which diffuses across the very narrow gap and stimulates the next axon to transmit impulses. There is more than one transmitter substance, but the best known is called acetylcholine. There is clearly a need for rapid removal of the acetylcholine once it has been released into a synapse, otherwise it will continue indefinitely to stimulate the transmission of impulses along adjacent axons. Normally the enzyme acetylcholinesterase (AChE) catalyses its rapid breakdown, but organophosphorus insecticides can combine with this enzyme, and so prevent, or slow down, the breakdown of acetylcholine. This can obviously disrupt the normal integrated pattern of behaviour. It is possible to show, both by biochemical assays of enzyme activity and by histochemical techniques, that the severity of the symptoms of poisoning increases as the degree of enzyme inhibition increases. It can also be shown, not surprisingly, that inhibition of some parts of the nervous system is more critical than of other parts. Animals regain their normal amounts of AChE once exposure has stopped, and it is usually presumed that there are no long-lasting effects. This may well be correct, and there is no particular reason to suppose otherwise, but it cannot be taken entirely for granted. A lot is still unknown about the metabolism of organophosphorus insecticides and even less is known about the biological effects and persistence of their metabolites.

Organophosphorus insecticides are not just specific inhibitors of AChE. They can inhibit a whole range of esterases, including the closely related cholinesterases, and other enzymes such as the ali-esterases. We do not know the precise importance to the animal for each of all these enzymes, and it was suggested at one time that these insecticides affected insects not by inhibition of AChE but by inhibition of an ali-esterase, in part because the ali-esterase was more easily inhibited. This suggestion has since been shown to be false, but we still do not know what is the effect of this ali-esterase inhibition.

Sometimes the effects are obvious. It has been known for a long time that some organophosphorus insecticides paralyse the limbs, especially the hind limbs. This results from inhibition of another, related, enzyme, which then causes damage to the structure of the membranes around the axons.

So we have with the organophosphorus insecticides a slight change of emphasis in the idea of the site of action. The primary lesion occurs in a group of enzymes, of which the most important is AChE, but other enzymes, in other sites, can also be affected.

One practical use is made of this inhibition of enzymes related to AChE. It would be exceedingly difficult to measure the degree of AChE inhibition in the synapses of industrial workers and others at risk from organophosphorus insecticides. It is therefore common

practice to assess the degree of exposure by measuring the cholinesterase activity of the blood. This is assumed to be a good index of
AChE activity, and it has been adequate for instances of relatively
severe poisoning, but some recent work by K. W. Jager *et al* suggests
it may be too insensitive to detect lesser effects. They examined
thirty-six workers who helped to manufacture and formulate these
insecticides, and found that about half of them had impaired nerve
and muscle function, although their blood cholinesterase activity
was unaffected. Muscle fibres responded less effectively to stimulation
by the nerve. We do not know whether this is a direct result of
AChE inhibition, or the result of another lesion, but it does illustrate
the difficulties of detecting sublethal effects. We will examine these
difficulties in more detail in Chapter six.

There has been considerable emphasis in this chapter on the
chemistry of insecticides. Chemical studies, especially analytical
results and methods, are an essential part of most pollution studies.
It was analytical problems which led to the discovery that another
class of pollutants was widespread in the environment. To comprehend how this came about, we must first consider briefly how residues
of organochlorine insecticides are measured.

Analysis, for any element or compound, can always be considered
under three headings. Firstly the element or compound may have to
be extracted from the sample. For organochlorines, this usually
means, with animal tissue, grinding up the tissue and treating with
reagents in such a way that the insecticide residues pass into a suitable
solvent, commonly hexane. This will leave behind the gross debris
and water-soluble compounds, but the extract will still contain many
fat-soluble compounds besides the organochlorine residues. Some of
these other compounds would interfere with the measurement of
insecticide residues, so a second 'clean-up' stage then removes as
much as possible of these interfering compounds without losing much,
or any, of the residues one is interested in. The details of the 'clean-
up' process will vary very much according to the type of sample, what
one is hoping to measure, and how much of it one expects to find.
The smaller the amount of residue, the more rigorous the 'clean-up'.
Finally one detects and measures the organochlorine insecticide
residues present in the 'cleaned-up' extract from the original sample.
The standard method is to inject a small amount of this extract into a
gas–liquid chromatograph. Essentially, what happens is that the
solvent and solutes are heated so that they vapourise. There is a
continuous stream of an inert gas which then carries the vapourised
compounds from the injected extract along a column, which is
packed with an inert solid coated with a non-volatile solvent.
Different gaseous compounds from the injected sample are retarded

to different degrees by the solvent as they pass along the column. Each compound travels along the column at its own characteristic speed, and so they become separated. So it is possible to measure the retention time, or time needed for each compound to travel the length of the column. Columns are commonly a few feet long, and retention times are usually measured in minutes. Thus the column achieves a final separation of compounds before they reach the detector. The detector for organochlorine insecticides is commonly a tritium cathode, that emits electrons to the anode, and the current is measured. Compounds such as DDT trap some of these electrons, and this decreases the current: hence the name electron-capture detector. The more DDT, the more the current decreases. In practice one obtains a chromatogram (Fig. 2-2), an ink line traced on moving

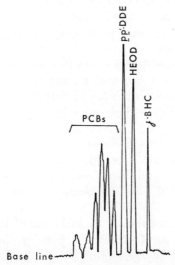

Fig. 2-2. Chromatogram for organochlorine residues in the liver of a barn owl (*Tyto alba*). Reproduced by courtesy of Mr M. C. French

graph paper by a pen that is linked to the detector and which changes its position as the current changes. The chromatogram consists of a base-line, which is the measure of the current when no detectable compounds are passing through, with a series of peaks, whose height and area indicate, by comparison with standard solutions, the amount of compound present. The base-line indicates how effective the 'clean-up' has been. Ideally, when no interfering substances are present, the base-line will be dead straight. In practice there are invariably some deviations in the base-line, and the magnitude of these deviations, or 'noise', limits the sensitivity, because the peak

c

produced by a compound cannot be measured unless it is greater than the background variation in the base-line.

This technique has several outstanding advantages. In particular, it is very sensitive, and it will detect several residues of interest at the same time. But it does not identify each residue unequivocally. Each peak is identified by its retention time, and one already knows, by injection of standard solutions, the retention times of the residues one wants to measure. So one presumes that if a sample produces a peak with the same retention time as *pp'*-DDT, it is *pp'*-DDT. It is possible however that another compound could have the same or a sufficiently similar retention time, and so be confused with *pp'*-DDT. This is not usually a problem with experimental material, where the control undosed animals help to confirm the identity. If there is sufficient residue in a specimen from the field, other techniques can be used to confirm the identity of the compound, but these methods are usually less sensitive. The mass spectrometer can be used, and is very sensitive, but this instrument is not yet generally available in analytical laboratories.

The electron-capture detector was first described by J. E. Lovelock and S. R. Lipsky in 1960, and during the first few years of use analysts in several laboratories found that chromatograms contained unidentified peaks. Often these were ignored, because they did not interfere too seriously with the analysis of known residues, but in 1966 it was reported that S. Jensen, in Sweden, had shown that these peaks in chromatograms from pike, eagle and human hair corresponded to polychlorobiphenyl compounds (PCBs). They are now known to be probably as ubiquitous in wildlife specimens as is DDE.

We discussed the conversion of DDT to PCB earlier on. Industrially, PCBs are manufactured by passing chlorine through biphenyl, which is a liquid, until the final product contains the desired percentage by weight of chlorine. The most widely used products contain from 42% to 60% chlorine. Unfortunately, the analysis of these products is not easy. A PCB of which chlorine constitutes 42% of the total weight will contain, on average, three chlorine atoms per molecule. But some molecules may contain fewer, down to none, and other molecules may contain up to the maximum number, of ten chlorine atoms. Furthermore, except for a molecule with either no or ten chlorine atoms, several or many isomers are possible. Altogether there are over 200 possible isomers, so that any industrial PCB is a mixture of many compounds. Thus the chromatogram of any particular PCB consists of a characteristic 'fingerprint' of a set of peaks of specific retention times and relative heights. Once there has been an opportunity for loss or conversion of these compounds, in wildlife specimens or in the physical environment, then the pattern of peaks will change, until it becomes impossible to identify the original PCB. For example, the PCBs with few chlorine atoms appear to disappear from wildlife specimens relatively rapidly. Few specific PCBs are available in standard solution, so that their recognition in specimens can become very difficult.

PCBs have many industrial uses, which include paints and varnishes, sealers in water-proofing compounds, printing inks, adhesives, hydraulic fluids, cutting oils and transformers. They have certainly been manufactured since the 1930s, and it is estimated that the total us production for 1957–1971 was about 360,000 metric tons. This was probably half of the world's total production. There has probably been several times as much DDT manufactured (Fig. 2-1), so it was of interest that G. R. Harvey *et al* found more than twenty times as much PCB in the surface water of the North Atlantic as of all DDT residues combined. It is not possible to be more precise about the ratio of PCB to DDT because the DDT residues were below the limit of detection. The simplest explanation is that PCB is much more persistent than are DDT residues. One might be tempted to suggest that some of the PCB comes, not from industrial sources, but from conversion of DDT in the atmosphere by ultraviolet radiation. One objection is that, in the laboratory at least, irradiation produced PCBs with two, three or four chlorine atoms, whereas molecules of PCB in the environment are usually said to contain rather more chlorine atoms.

There was initially some scepticism that PCBs were widespread. Unlike insecticides, they are not usually released deliberately into the environment, although considerable amounts must eventually be released in sewage sludge, burning of waste products and so forth. PCBs are however, like the organochlorine insecticides, chemically stable, soluble in fats and oils, and of low solubility in water, and they were soon found to be widespread in wildlife. For example, a survey was conducted from Monks Wood into the amounts of PCBs found in bird livers from various parts of Great Britain (Fig. 2-3). One hundred and thirty livers were analysed from birds of prey. This cannot be regarded as a random sample, because these birds were found dead or dying, but the map does demonstrate that PCBs are present in relatively large amounts from diverse habitats throughout the country, and are not restricted to samples taken near industrial areas. Similar work from Europe and the usa shows that PCBs are indeed widespread in the environment.

My first acquaintance with PCBs was entirely unexpected and, at the time, baffling. I had designed an experiment to test the biological

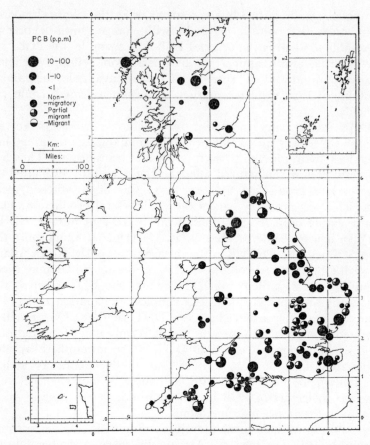

Fig. 2-3. Survey of PCB residues found in the livers of terrestrial predatory wild birds. The livers were taken from birds found dead or dying
during 1966–1968. (Data from I. Prestt, D. J. Jefferies & N. W. Moore,
1970.)

effects of dieldrin on some caterpillars. This was a controlled
laboratory experiment, and in due course my colleague, M. C. French,
our analyst at Monks Wood, ran cleaned-up extracts from the
caterpillars through a gas–liquid chromatograph to measure the
amounts of dieldrin. Normally chromatograms from control,
undosed, caterpillars gave a reasonably smooth base-line, but in this
particular experiment there were many large peaks, which entirely
masked the peak for dieldrin from dosed caterpillars. Eventually we
had to abandon all results from this experiment, because we did not
know what these compounds were, or how the caterpillars had got
them. Some time later M. C. French saw some of the first chromatograms for PCBs, and instantly recognised the pattern of peaks found

in the caterpillars. Decorators had been revarnishing some of the exterior woodwork at the time of this experiment, varnishes often contain PCBs, and presumably the caterpillars had picked up some PCB from this activity, although they were in a room with no open windows, and whose only door opened into the middle of the building.

Great care is sometimes needed to ensure that samples are not inadvertently contaminated. Jensen *et al* sampled plankton from a boat in Stockholm harbour. Samples taken from astern of the boat contained more than twenty times as much PCB as those taken with nets attached to the bowsprit. The boat's hull had been painted about two months earlier, and PCBs from the paint were contaminating the water.

These two experiences suggest that, because PCBs have such diverse uses, they can readily escape into the environment. There is still a lot to be found out about PCBs, but it is noteworthy that these compounds had been in the environment for at least two decades before we discovered, by chance, that they were there. It is a nice question whether they have adverse effects on wildlife, and we will return to this theme in Chapter seven.

Monsanto Chemicals are the sole manufacturers of PCBs in the UK and USA. When they realised how widespread these compounds are in the environment they withdrew them from all uses where there was much likelihood of their being released into the environment. This partial ban started in 1970 in the USA, and early in 1971 in the UK. It will be interesting to see what effect this enlightened reaction has, both on amounts in the environment and on other manufacturers of these compounds.

3

The Peregrine Falcon, and Other Birds

There has been fierce controversy in Britain about the effects that pesticides may have had on wildlife. This argument has focussed largely on predatory birds, and was stimulated by a rather odd chain of events.

Many people fly racing pigeons. It is one of the normal hazards of this activity that sometimes a bird fails to return home from a race. There are many possible reasons for such losses, but by 1960 there were complaints that the number of peregrine falcons was increasing, and that they were killing more racing pigeons than hitherto. There was little or no direct evidence for this assertion, but it could not be positively dismissed as untrue. The peregrine (*Falco peregrinus*), the largest falcon native to Great Britain, feeds almost entirely on live birds, which it captures in flight. The peregrine's principal prey species, south of the Scottish Highlands, is the domestic pigeon, although it can and does prey on a wide range of other birds too.

So, in response to these complaints, D. A. Ratcliffe, of the Nature Conservancy, started a survey, in conjunction with the British Trust for Ornithology, to see whether there had been a recent increase in the numbers and distribution of breeding pairs of the peregrine falcon. Fortunately, this is one of the few wildlife species for which we have extensive and reasonably accurate figures of population size in the past. In part this is because of the bird's use in falconry, in part because the peregrine has a relatively small, and stable, population. The nest, or eyrie, is often made in the same spot year after year, usually on a steep rock face. This need for a steep rock face does in fact limit their distribution, and when a pair disappear from a territory they are usually soon replaced by another pair. Consequently the total number of breeding pairs appears to have been remarkably stable. For example, of forty-nine eyries which were recorded between the sixteenth and nineteenth centuries, forty-one were still occupied in 1930–1939. The Second World War illustrated this stability. There were about 700 pairs of peregrine in Great

36

Britain during the nineteen thirties. The Air Ministry virtually exterminated the species from southern England during the war so as to protect carrier pigeons. This control stopped in 1945, and the peregrine falcon rapidly recolonised many of its old haunts during the next five years.

Ratcliffe's survey showed, contrary to expectation, that there had been a recent, and rapid, decline in numbers again after the post-war recovery. This decline started in southern England, in about 1955, and then spread northwards all the way to parts of the Scottish Highlands. By 1962 51 % of all the known pre-war territories were deserted, and the figure was as high as 93 % for southern England. Examination of the pre-war data suggests that, in any one year, about 85 % of known territories should be occupied by breeding pairs. Furthermore, there were successful nestings in only 26 % of the occupied territories.

These findings clearly dismissed the complaints about predation of racing pigeons, but raised other questions. What was causing this rapid decline in numbers and lessened breeding success? Here we have a species whose numbers, so far as we can tell, remain very constant except when intensively persecuted. And now, in less than a decade, there had been a dramatic decline. Study of the factors which control population size is the keystone of animal ecology, and there is much that we do not yet understand about how these controls work. But we can review the likely possibilities for the peregrine.

Firstly, this might be a normal long term fluctuation of population size, caused perhaps by a change of climate. We do not know whether such a fluctuation has occurred before, because we only have adequate records for the number of breeding pairs from early in this century. However, this species is widespread throughout Eurasia and North America, and tolerates a wide range of conditions, and yet a similar decline in the number of peregrines occurred at about the same time in various parts of Europe and the USA. So climatic change is an unlikely explanation.

Secondly, a serious shortage of food could obviously reduce the population size. This has in fact occurred in many parts of the western Highlands and Islands of Scotland, where the main prey species is the red grouse (*Lagopus lagopus*). Grouse feed principally on heather. The heather has been overgrazed by sheep and deer, and has often been burnt indiscriminately, so that during the last sixty years or so the amount and luxuriance of the heather has declined. Concomitantly the number of grouse and of peregrine has declined because of food shortage. Elsewhere in Britain there is no evidence for a shortage of food for peregrines.

Thirdly, the decline could be caused by disease. The natural incidence, and types, of disease that affect peregrines are unknown, but it seems unlikely that an epidemic of this size and severity could have been overlooked.

Fourthly, these birds have always been liable to human interference. Game-keepers shoot them, collectors take their eggs, other human activities may incidentally disturb them. There is no reason to suppose however that these influences have increased materially since before the war.

In brief, the 'natural' factors that influence survival can be classified as climate, food, other animals—including organisms that cause disease, and a place in which to live. There is no good evidence to suggest that a change in any of these 'natural' factors has caused the rapid decline in the number of peregrine falcons.

This conclusion leaves few reasonable alternative explanations. In fact a pollutant is the only one that readily comes to mind. When and where such a pollutant occurs in the environment would presumably be correlated with when and where the numbers and breeding success dropped. This argument rules out radioactive isotopes from atomic and thermo-nuclear explosions. The degree to which these isotopes are deposited in Great Britain is highest in the north and west of Great Britain, where the peregrine has been relatively unaffected. There are however many other possible candidates: one aspect of the current technological revolution is the enormous increase during the past twenty-five years in the number and amounts of novel synthetic compounds. Some of these compounds persist for a considerable time in the physical environment. For the moment it is sufficient to state that, at that stage in the investigation, organochlorine insecticides were considered as possible candidates, if only because, at that time, they were the only pollutants whose effects on wildlife had received much attention in this country. Unlike many other persistent pollutants, they were virtually nonexistent until the Second World War, when DDT, the first of the organochlorine insecticides, was used in large quantities. After the war their use in agriculture developed rapidly, and many tons were soon being used each year. Residues of several organochlorine insecticides were found when peregrine eggs were analysed. The amounts present were in general greatest in those areas where the greatest decrease in peregrine numbers had occurred (Table 3-1), although there were so few birds left in some areas that none of the few available eggs were taken for analysis. The major compound detected was DDE, a conversion product of DDT that is commonly found in animals. All eggs contained either DDE or HEOD, and the great majority of eggs contained both. So there was a correlation between the concentration of organochlorine insecticide residues and

Table 3-1. Analyses of peregrine falcon eggs collected during the years 1963–1969. Amounts are expressed as concentrations in the fresh eggs, in parts per million. The arithmetic means and the range of concentrations found are shown. tr indicates a trace. (Data from D. A. Ratcliffe, 1970.)

Region	Number of eggs analysed	DDE (a derivative of DDT)	HEOD (the active principle of dieldrin)	Heptachlor epoxide	Total organochlorine residues
East and Central Highlands of Scotland	16	3.25 tr–8.6	0.29 tr–1.6	0.28 0–3.0	4.01 tr–14.95
Rest of Britain	42	13.67 0.2–33.0	0.57 0–2.6	0.54 0–4.3	15.16 0.2–36.1

the decline in peregrine numbers. These results were very suggestive, but it was a far cry from being able to say that the residues caused the decline.

If some or all of these residues did reduce the number of peregrine falcons, how did they do it? Two facts make this question particularly difficult to answer. Firstly, we are dealing with something that has already happened, so that we cannot observe the process while it actually takes place. Secondly, it is impracticable to use the peregrine falcon for experiments. This bird could not, with any reasonable amount of resources, be bred in captivity in sufficient numbers. However, Ratcliffe had already noted the first clue before any question about pesticides had arisen.

Until about 1950, each breeding pair of falcons laid one clutch of eggs each year, which contained almost invariably either three or four eggs. The mean number of eggs per clutch was 3.5. These eggs are not usually replaced unless lost early on. The mean number of fledged young used to be 2.5. The other egg was usually lost either because the embryo did not hatch (infertility of egg or death of embryo) or because the young chick died in the nest. Only 4% of clutches had any broken eggs. During the period 1951–1966 the number of clutches with broken eggs rose to 39%. Direct human or other interference was a most unlikely explanation, and the phenomenon was inexplicable when first recorded. We do not know precisely when eggs started to break more often. It is well authenticated from 1951 onwards, but could have started a couple of years earlier. Certainly, this reduced breeding success was not the immediate cause of a population decrease, because numbers did not start to decline until, at the earliest, five years later. So there are now three questions. What part, if any, did residues of organochlorine insecticides play in reducing the population of peregrines, and in increasing the frequency of broken eggs in the eyries? And what connection is there between lower reproductive success and smaller population size?

Ratcliffe decided next to measure the eggshell thickness of eggs which had been collected in known years, to see whether the increase in egg breakage coincided with a decrease in eggshell thickness. The measurements had to be made without damaging the eggs, so an index of eggshell thickness was used:

$$\frac{\text{eggshell weight}}{\text{egg length} \times \text{egg breadth}}$$

This index has been calculated for eggs collected between 1901 and 1969, and it dropped abruptly during 1947 and 1948 by, on average, 19.1% (Fig. 3-1). The pre-war value appears to have been very stable—there was no significant difference in the index for forty-nine

British and continental peregrine eggs collected in 1845–1865. More-over, only since 1947 have there been geographical variations within Great Britain in this index: eggs from inland areas of the central and eastern Scottish Highlands have shown a decrease of only 4.4 %. There was no evidence for any change in egg size. This reduced index

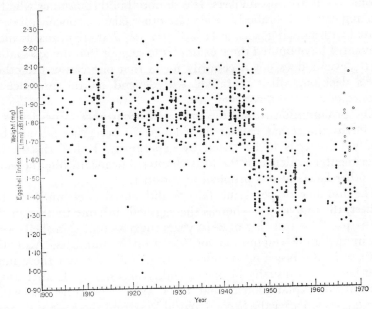

Fig. 3-1. Changes from 1901–1969 of the eggshell index for the peregrine falcon in Great Britain. ◯, eggshells from the central and east Scottish Highlands; ●, eggshells from other districts. (Data from D. A. Ratcliffe, 1970.)

value was caused, at least in large part, by a thinning of the shell. The shell, which is 90 % calcium carbonate, may also have become less dense.

These results were most illuminating. Eggs with thinner and less dense shells are presumably weaker mechanically, and this could explain why the rate of egg breakage had increased. Furthermore, these observations suggest an experimental approach.

All the evidence presented so far consists of observations that changes in one factor are associated with changes in another factor. This is a perfectly valid approach, and has of course, under the name of epidemiology, been used in medical research for a very long time. However, its limitations must be realised.

For example, there has been much controversy in recent years about the effects of smoking. We know that for moderate cigarette smokers the death rate from lung cancer is about ten times as high as the rate for non-smokers, and the rate increases to twenty or thirty times for heavy smokers. Most people now accept that smoking can cause cancer, although one cannot eliminate the possibility that some individuals are genetically predisposed to both smoking and lung cancer. Smokers are also about twice as likely to die from coronary thrombosis as are non-smokers. It is doubtful in this instance whether smoking causes thrombosis—there are other factors, conceivably correlated with smoking, such as lack of exercise, that are probably more relevant. I have quoted these examples to suggest that the association of two events does not necessarily mean that one causes the other. One's decision, albeit tentative, will depend on the presence or absence of corroborative evidence.

The presumption is that the increased occurrence of pesticides in the environment has caused the changes in peregrine falcons, but ideally this needs to be tested by experiment. I shall discuss the experimental evidence in the next chapter, but meanwhile there are two other facets of this problem to consider.

The number of peregrine falcons did not decline until, at the earliest, the mid-1950s, whereas the eggshells became thinner in the late 1940s. This time lag of 8–10 years suggests that thin shells were not immediately responsible for the drop in numbers. Also, the decrease in the breeding population was so abrupt that there must have been an unusually heavy mortality of adult birds after 1955. The current explanation is that DDT and BHC came into widespread use soon after the Second World War, and these are presumed to have initiated thinner eggshells. The cyclodiene insecticides then came into widespread agricultural use after 1955, especially as seed dressings. These too are presumed to have caused thinner eggshells, but, in addition, it is believed that they caused the decline in numbers. Dieldrin was used extensively as a seed dressing for both autumn and spring sown cereal seed. There were some notorious incidents of birds, especially pigeons, found dead and dying in the spring after eating dressed seed, and it is suggested that a peregrine falcon which ate two or three heavily contaminated pigeons would itself die. The already existing decline in breeding success then helped to prevent a return to normal numbers.

The other facet is this. If pesticides have caused peregrine falcons to lay eggs with thinner eggshells, one might expect to find the same effect in other species too. This is in fact the case. The most extreme example must be the brown pelican (*Pelecanus occidentalis*), which occurs in the USA. A colony of this bird on Anacapa Island, off the Californian coast, laid eggs in 1969 which were only half as thick as those laid before 1943. These shells were in fact so weak that many were soft.

One of the most interesting examples is the golden eagle (*Aquila chrysaetos*), which, in the British Isles, occurs principally in the Scottish Highlands. Birds in eastern and central Scotland have shown little change in the last few decades, but in western Scotland the eggshell index declined by 9.9% after the war, and breeding success dropped too. This difference between regions is correlated with differences in feeding habit. In western Scotland eagles feed habitually on sheep carrion, but they do not in central and eastern Scotland, where there is a good supply of wild prey, and where in some areas there are few or no sheep anyway. J. D. Lockie and D. A. Ratcliffe suggested that eagles were acquiring significant amounts of dieldrin from sheep carrion—sheep were dipped annually in dieldrin as a protection against blowfly. Home-killed mutton, analysed by the Government Chemist's Laboratory, was found to contain up to 10 ppm dieldrin in the fat. Dieldrin was banned from use in sheep dips from the start of 1966, and the residues in mutton fat then declined:

Year	Number of samples	Residues in mutton fat (ppm)	
		Mean	Range
1964	128	0.8	0.0–12.4
1965	107	1.1	0.0– 8.2
1966	101	0.44	0.0– 5.3
1967	76	0.24	0.0– 8.0
1968	77	0.21	0.0–10.4
1969	53	0.04	0.0– 0.6
1970	35	0.01	0.0– 0.2

The relative slowness of the decline was attributed to the continued use by farmers of old stocks of dieldrin. There were correlated changes in the egg residues, and breeding success, of the golden eagle in western Scotland (data from J. D. Lockie, D. A. Ratcliffe & R. Balharry, 1969):

Period	Number of nests with eggs	% of nests from which young flew	Number of eggs analysed	Mean dieldrin conc. in eggs (ppm)
1963–1965	39	31	48	0.86
1966–1968	45	69	23	0.34

During all of this period eagles bred very successfully in eastern Scotland, with young flying from 70–80% of the nests, and with low egg residues, which never exceeded 0.1 ppm dieldrin.

Altogether Ratcliffe examined eggs from 17 species of British birds, and found that many of them had started to lay thinner egg-shells since the Second World War. The results are summarised briefly below:

Species	% change in eggshell index	
Peregrine	−19	
Sparrowhawk	−17	
Merlin	−13	
Shag	−12	
Golden eagle (from western Scotland)	−10	significant change
Hobby	−5	
Rook	−5	
Kestrel	−5	
Carrion crow	−5	
Golden plover	−2	
Kittiwake	−1	
Raven	−1	
Guillemot	0	
Buzzard	0	no significant change
Razorbill	+1	
Greenshank	+1	
Black-headed gull	+1	

In general, the greater the drop in the eggshell index the higher the concentration of organochlorine residues. In none of these species had the eggs become smaller since 1945: the eggshells had become thinner.

It has been a matter for speculation as to the precise connection between thinner eggshells and increased incidence of egg breakage. Thinner eggshells will be weaker, and so less able to withstand the normal stresses and strains within the nest. There have also been suggestions that the parent birds deliberately destroy their eggs, either because the pesticides have induced aberrant behaviour, or in an attempt to rectify a shortage of calcium, which again has been induced by the pesticide, and which is expressed by the thinner eggshells. However, it has been reported for the osprey that the results stem from changes in the egg, although the full details have not yet been published. Ospreys in the Chesapeake Bay area have been flourishing, whereas those in New England have been declining. P. Spitzer transferred eggs from the failing osprey population in New England to the nests of a flourishing population in the Chesapeake Bay area, and vice versa. The eggs were unaffected by the change, and those that were transferred from New England produced as few viable young around Chesapeake Bay as would have been expected if they had remained in the original nests.

I have already referred to the difficulties of experimental work on peregrine falcons. However, one 'natural' experiment has occurred within the last decade. I have assumed so far that if these changes have been caused by pollutants, it is the organochlorine insecticides that

Table 3-2. The number of breeding pairs of peregrine falcons in Great Britain. (Data from D. A. Ratcliffe, 1972.)

Region	*1962* Number of territories examined	*1962* % occupied	*1971* Number of territories examined	*1971* % occupied
Southern England	73	7	92	11
Wales	88	22	141	18
Coastal territories in northern England and Scotland	155	65	220	46
Inland territories in northern England and Scotland	172	67	273	75
Total for Great Britain	488	49	726	47

are responsible. The amounts of organochlorine insecticide released into the environment in Great Britain have decreased since the mid-1960s, so one might expect the numbers of peregrine falcons to have increased again since then. Ratcliffe conducted a second survey of peregrine numbers in 1971 to test this presumption. In fact the results pointed to a rather confused situation. Table 3-2 compares results obtained in the two surveys. This comparison is complicated, because the surveys were not based on exactly the same eyries. The later survey was the more complete, when 90% of all known territories were examined. Strictly, results should only be compared for territories that were examined in both surveys. However, conclusions from such a more limited comparison are similar to those given here.

The two surveys gave similar results for southern England and Wales, with few territories occupied on either occasion. The territories in Scotland and the rest of England fall into two distinct categories—inland and coastal. A higher proportion of the inland territories was occupied in 1971, but, contrary to expectation, there had been a further decrease since 1962 in all the coastal territories except for southern Scotland. These results are anomalous: why hasn't the number of breeding pairs increased in the coastal territories? One would expect peregrines to recolonise their old haunts quite rapidly once the adverse effects of pollutants have diminished sufficiently.

Annual local censuses confirmed that these differences are not chance or random variations, but are consistent changes. For example, the population for inland territories in north-west England started to recover from the mid-1960s on, whereas the decline started in the mid-1960s in Orkney, and has continued ever since:

| | N.W. England | | Orkney | |
Year	Number of territories visited	% occupied by breeding pairs	Number of territories visited	% occupied by breeding pairs
1961	33	73	17	100
1962	33	45	24	96
1963	28	36	18	94
1964	27	37	16	63
1965	33	33	18	61
1966	27	33	22	55
1967	32	50	19	63
1968	28	61	14	57
1969	28	71	20	65
1970	30	70	19	68
1971	35	69	24	58

It has already been suggested that pesticides prevented the recovery of peregrine populations by their adverse effects on breeding success.

There are many possible criteria of success: the term is used here to indicate a pair of peregrines that lays and hatches a clutch of eggs. The figures for breeding success in 1971, like those for the numbers of breeding pairs, distinguish between coastal and inland territories (Table 3-3). Fewer coastal pairs of falcons bred successfully in 1971 than in 1962, whereas there was a marked improvement in inland areas. Ratcliffe suggests that pairs in coastal districts are now being affected by marine pollutants, acquired by feeding on sea birds. Certainly eggs from eyries on or near the coast contain on average several times as much PCB as those from inland districts, which suggests, not surprisingly, that such birds have a different type of exposure to pollutants.

This second survey produced one other surprising feature too. Eggshell thickness in 1971 was similar to that for the previous two decades, even though the residues of organochlorine insecticides were smaller. However, there are at least two reasons for interpreting such data with caution. Data from all of the analyses of eggs made during 1963–1969 suggest that although the eggshell index does decrease as the total content of organochlorine insecticides increases, once the concentration reaches about 5–10 ppm the index remains stable. So eggshells will not become thicker again until the amount of residues drops below this critical value. In addition, we have no reason to suppose that only organochlorine insecticides may thin eggshells. The effects of other pollutants have had a comparatively cursory investigation, but it has been found that both PCBs and mercury can sometimes thin eggshells.

Taken altogether, the field evidence does make a strong argument that pesticides did affect some bird populations in the 1950s and early 1960s. There was, as the current phrase has it, coincidence in both space and time between the occurrence of pesticides in the environment and the sublethal and lethal effects on bird populations. However, suggestive though it is, one must remember that this evidence is correlative. Results of the 1971 survey have produced anomalies in both the geographical pattern of recovery in numbers, and of the continued thinness of eggshells. These may be the results of other pollutants. My personal opinion, which is based on the experimental evidence described in the next chapter as well as on the field data, is that exposure to organochlorine insecticides did initiate the changes that have affected peregrine falcons, and that other pollutants such as PCBs are perhaps now involved too. We probably never will know for certain.

To my mind one of the most remarkable features of the whole incident is the way in which this species virtually disappeared from some parts of Great Britain without our realising it. This does under-

D

Table 3-3. The breeding success of peregrine falcons in Great Britain. (Data from D. A. Ratcliffe, 1972.)

Region	1962		1971	
	Number of occupied territories	% with hatched eggs	Number of occupied territories	% with hatched eggs
Southern England	5	40	10	50
Wales	19	16	26	19
Coastal territories in northern England and Scotland	101	48	101	42
Inland territories in northern England and Scotland	116	34	204	51
Total for Great Britain	241	38	341	46

line the need for adequate monitoring of the environment in order to avoid similar incidents in the future passing unnoticed until it is too late to do anything about them. The analytical results also show, regardless of what biological significance one attaches to them, that these compounds can concentrate to a remarkable degree in living organisms.

4

Thin Eggshells

The recent thinning of eggshells in wild birds was first reported by Ratcliffe in 1967. Since then, it has been shown that some populations of about forty species now lay eggs with shells thinner than they used to be. It has also been found that, in general, the more highly contaminated eggs tend to have the thinner shells. This association is true in particular for DDE, which is usually the most abundant organochlorine insecticide residue. Interpretation of such data can however be difficult. For example, amounts of DDE are often correlated with amounts of PCB. It is not suggested that the shells are thinner because of the pollutant present in the egg, but this is taken as an index of the amount of pollutant in the laying bird, which, it is thought, does cause thinner shells.

More than forty experiments to test the effects of pollutants on shell thickness have now been described: some of them suffer from a defect common with research into highly topical subjects—the emphasis appears to be more to get something published than to increase our understanding.

In general, gallinaceous species such as the domestic hen, pheasant and quail appear to be less affected by any particular level of organochlorine compounds in their diet than are other species. Falcons appear to be amongst the most susceptible. Rarely are tissues analysed for residues, so we don't know whether this means that gallinaceous species get rid of their pollutants more quickly, or are less susceptible to amounts in the body.

Experimental birds are usually dosed by mixing the pollutant into their diet. The amount of pollutant ingested is then the product of the concentration in the diet and of the amount of contaminated food that is eaten. Unfortunately, the amount of food that the birds eat has been noted in very few of the published experiments. This may not matter very much if food consumption is unaffected by the pollutant. In fact, it has been found several times that organochlorine insecticides can affect, and usually reduce, food consumption to a considerable degree when there is no other food available. One might suppose that the insecticide made the food less palatable, but the same effect has also been found with pheasants given dieldrin in capsules, and with pigeons fed DDT in capsules. This detail is very important, because reduced food consumption can cause thinner eggshells. For example, A. S. Cooke fed chickens on a normal diet for five days, starved them for the next two, and then resumed feeding them. Eggs laid on the second day of starvation had shells sixteen per cent thinner than usual, and shells were twenty-two per cent thinner on the next day. They regained their normal thickness by the twelfth day of the experiment.

Of course, if insecticides cause thinner shells because they reduce food consumption, then not only have we demonstrated that they can cause thinning, but also how they do it. If residues act in laboratory experiments by reducing food intake, we would then need to confirm that residues acquired with food in the field also act in this way. It could well be that wild terrestrial animals acquire most of their residues in a small part of their total food intake, and that total food consumption is unaffected. If this were the situation, then experiments that purport to demonstrate that pollutants cause thinner egg-shells would be irrelevant to field situations. In fact, so far as the evidence goes, it looks as though food consumption is not affected except by relatively high concentrations of organochlorine insecticide, but we still await the definitive experiment in which a pollutant is administered, residues are comparable to those found in field specimens, food consumption is unaffected, and eggshells are thinner.

S. N. Wiemeyer and R. D. Porter, at the Patuxent Wildlife Research Center, in the USA, fed twelve pairs of American kestrels (*Falco sparverius*) on a diet with 2.8 ppm DDE in minced meat. This diet was started at the end of March, 1968, when the females were just about to lay eggs, and it was continued until eggs were next laid in 1969. Twelve control pairs were kept on a similar diet, but without added DDE. Where possible, the first egg from each clutch was collected and the shell thickness measured. The results (Table 4-1)

Table 4-1. The effect of 2.8 ppm DDE in the diet on the thickness of eggshells of the American kestrel (*Falco sparverius*). Thicknesses, with standard errors, are given in microns. (Data from S. N. Wiemeyer & R. D. Porter, 1970.)

	1968	*1969*
Control birds	188 ± 7	184 ± 8
Dosed birds	186 ± 5	168 ± 4

show clearly that there was no significant change in the controls—the shells in 1969 were 2.1% thinner than in 1968, but this can be attributed to chance variations. The dosed birds too, in 1968, were not affected, but by 1969, after a year's exposure to DDE, the shells were 9.7% thinner. Comparisons of eggs laid by the same birds in both years showed that such a large decrease would happen by chance less than once in a thousand similar experiments, so one can conclude that the DDE caused the thinner eggshells.

This would appear to be a straightforward convincing experiment, even though, as we have already seen, lack of information on food consumption makes interpretation of some aspects rather difficult. But B. C. Switzer *et al* made 'a critical review' of this paper, and concluded that the evidence did not show that DDE caused shell thinning. They argued from the range of values found within each group of eggshells:

	1968	*1969*
Control birds	130–210 microns	130–210 microns
Dosed birds	165–203 microns	153–185 microns

They pointed out, correctly, that the thinnest eggshells in both years, 130 microns thick, were laid by the control group. They deduced, incorrectly, that this nullified the differences between the mean thicknesses. This criticism does of course ignore the means and standard errors (shown in Table 4-1), which are a far more relevant test of the difference between two groups than is the difference between the lowest values found within the two groups. It also ignores the experimental design, which allowed one to test for differences in individual birds in the two years.

This criticism has no intrinsic significance, except to add two more references—one for the criticism, one for the rebuttal—to the files of those interested in these matters. I quote it to illustrate a problem that is common in scientific research of immediate public interest. Those in research are, or should be, quite capable of defending themselves against ill-based criticism. And fellow scientists who are professionally interested should be capable of reaching their own conclusions. But interested laymen have two handicaps. Firstly, they may not be technically competent to judge the intricacies at issue; I have deliberately chosen a very simple example. Furthermore, they will probably be unaware of much of the relevant information. This can make life perplexing. Another ill-founded criticism of the experimental work on shell thinning, by W. Hazeltine, was summarised in '*The Times*', within a week of its first publication, with the title 'Pesticides: exploding the DDE myth', and started off 'The belief that DDT residues make birds' egg shells dangerously thin is a myth'. Perhaps all I am really saying is that one should never accept any information without question, and always retain some degree of scepticism, even when the source appears to be unimpeachable. Personally I tend to regard with suspicion any criticism or defence that cannot be put in terms that I can understand.

Wiemeyer and Porter also analysed their experimental eggs for DDE residues (Table 4-2). Controls laid eggs with a fairly constant

Table 4–2. Mean concentrations and standard errors (in ppm) for DDE residues found in eggs of the American kestrel (*Falco sparverius*). (Data from S. N. Wiemeyer & R. D. Porter, 1970.)

	1968	*1969*
Control birds	0.62±0.05	0.71±0.05
Dosed birds	3.09±0.45	32.4±2.78

low degree of contamination, whilst the dosed birds were, after a year's exposure, laying eggs with rather more than twice the concentration of DDE found in peregrine falcons (Table 3-1). These residue figures are very useful because they enable us to relate, albeit imperfectly, the results of laboratory experiments to events in the field. The relationship between exposure and residues is very important, and we will consider it in the next chapter. The residue figures do help us to decide whether experimental exposures are of the same order of magnitude as those encountered in the field, although qualifications include possible differences between species and effects of other variables. We know at present very little about either. Again, few of the experimental studies so far give residue data.

Despite the weak links in the argument, many workers have tacitly assumed that insecticides do thin eggshells, and much attention has been focused on possible mechanisms. Rather surprisingly, physiological and biochemical speculations and experiments were rife for several years before any details were published of any morphological examinations. I shall reverse the historical order, and discuss first the normal eggshell structure.

Most of our knowledge of eggshell structure relates to the domestic chicken, and most of what follows is based on this species. We have no reason to suppose that other species of bird differ in any important respects, but this is, to a large extent, an assumption.

Once an egg is released from the ovary, it passes down the oviduct, where the yolk is covered first by a thick layer of albumen (egg-white) and then by membranes. The egg then passes into the shell gland, where, within the next twenty hours, most if not all of the hard outer eggshell is deposited. About ninety-five % of this shell is mineral matter (i.e. inorganic compounds), and of this mineral matter more than ninety-five% is calcium carbonate, deposited in its most stable crystalline form, calcite. So the eggshell consists almost entirely of calcite. But the small amount of organic matter is important. Some of this organic matter (mucoprotein) occurs in distinct concentrations, which are spaced fairly regularly on the out-side of the egg membrane, and which are called mammillary cores (Fig. 4-1). These cores act as nuclei about which the first calcite crystals are deposited, and these deposits grow predominantly out-wards from the membrane, to form the mammillary layer, until they coalesce with the adjacent cones. They then grow as separate

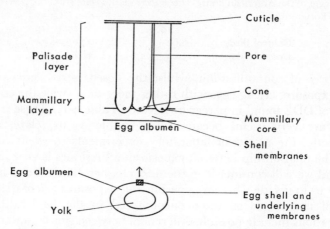

Fig. 4-1. Diagrammatic cross section of bird's eggshell

contiguous columns, to form the palisade layer. A loose analogy can be provided by visualising a group of closely packed stalagmites growing up from the floor of a cave. Occasionally the calcite columns do not coalesce, but leave pores. The calcified shell is permeated by a continuous organic matrix, which consists largely of mucoprotein. Although this matrix is quantitatively very minor, it may be very important—matrix deposition precedes calcite deposition, and this matrix may control shell development. Finally the outside of the palisade layer is covered, in the chicken eggshell, by an **organic** cuticle. Some species have an additional, superficial, cover.

Two West German workers, H. K. Erben and G. Krampitz, pub-lished details of the first morphological examination in 1971. They used an electron microscope to study the ultrastructure of two shells from the colony of brown pelicans on Anacapa Island. These shells were only 200 and 360 microns thick, compared to a shell 590 microns thick from an unaffected population. The mammillary layer was relatively normal, but the palisade layer was thinner, which suggests a deficiency in the supply of calcium carbonate. The normal orientation of calcite crystals in the palisade layer was disrupted, there was an increased number of globular inclusions, and the organic matter had a different chemical composition. These thin shells had a cuticle and cover, so it is unlikely that the eggs were laid prematurely. Rather, one of the normal physiological processes must have been disturbed.

Many mechanisms have been suggested for shell thinning, with various degrees of experimental support. These suggestions can arbitrarily be divided into four categories: reduced supplies of calcium or of carbonate, other changes in the eggshell, or changes in the laying bird. I will discuss one of the more prominent theories, which may serve to illustrate the possible complexities when one tries to unravel mechanisms. Carbonate for eggshells is now believed to come from metabolic carbon dioxide, most of which is of course excreted via the lungs in the breath. A minor part of the carbon dioxide that is dissolved in the tissue fluids combines with water to form carbonic acid, some of which then dissociates into hydrogen and bicarbonate ions:

$$CO_2 + H_2O \underset{\substack{\text{carbonic} \\ \text{anhydrase}}}{\rightleftharpoons} H_2CO_3 \rightleftharpoons H^+ + HCO_3^-$$

Carbon dioxide combines very slowly with water, so that, in normal physiological conditions, the equilibrium concentration of carbonic acid would not be approached. In practice this reaction is accelerated by the enzyme carbonic anhydrase. If this enzyme were inhibited, there would be less carbonic acid, and therefore a shortage of bicarbonate ions from which to form calcium carbonate. It is known that sulphanilamide, which inhibits carbonic anhydrase, does immediately reduce shell thickness, and this is probably because of the enzyme inhibition. It is then superficially attractive to suggest that organochlorine insecticides thin eggshells in the same way. It is true that carbonic anhydrase is water soluble, whereas the insecticides are fat soluble, but it has been found that these insecticides can bind with soluble proteins.

Experiments have been made both *in vitro* and *in vivo* to see whether enzyme inhibition occurs. Some of the early *in vitro* experiments apparently showed that addition of DDT to a solution of non-avian carbonic anhydrase reduced the enzyme's activity, possibly by inhibition, but it was later shown that, in the experimental conditions used, the DDT had precipitated out and occluded some of the enzyme at the same time. However, work has since been quoted to show that solutions of avian carbonic anhydrase are truly inhibited by DDT. Of course, the fact that DDT will inhibit a solution of this enzyme does not mean that such inhibition will necessarily occur in the whole animal. At the simplest, DDT may be unable to reach the enzyme. There are a few observations, of uncertain validity, on dosed intact birds to suggest that insecticides may reduce the carbonic anhydrase activity of the shell gland.

Cooke argues, from a detailed discussion of possible mechanisms, that probably there is not one dominant cause, but several potential mechanisms, and that species, condition of the bird and environmental conditions all help determine the degree to which each mechanism is involved. Obviously much more work will need to be done on this topic before we can reach any firm conclusions. The problem is a fascinating one for biochemists and physiologists, but it may seem a somewhat esoteric subject to those who are not especially interested in such matters. There are however at least two good practical reasons for such studies. It would enable us to decide the relative importance of pollutants and other environmental factors for shell thinning, and it would help us to predict, once we knew the sites of action, how much pollution is needed to thin eggshells.

5

Exposure and Residues

There is a widely held view, which has a considerable amount of truth in it, that a subject only matures as a science when it becomes quantitative. To some extent of course it depends on one's definition of a science. Personally I like to define science as those activities with which scientists amuse themselves, and certainly many scientists have a predilection for using numbers whenever possible.

In pollution studies, often the only hard datum available is the amount of pollutant, or residue, found by chemical analysis to be present in a body, organ or tissue. The amount of residue present is usually expressed as a concentration: so much weight of pollutant per unit weight of specimen e.g. parts per million (ppm), or equivalent expressions such as milligrams per kilogram (mg/kg). Smaller amounts may be expressed as parts per billion, which means parts per thousand million in the USA, and parts per million million in Great Britain.

The interest in residues is two-fold. The size of the residue gives some indication of past exposure. It can also give some indication of whether exposure to that pollutant is likely to have affected the organism. I shall discuss the first topic in this chapter, and the second topic in the next chapter.

Before we go any further, I must just mention a few details about the measurement of residue concentrations. Firstly, there are several ways of measuring the body weight. Most frequently it is measured as fresh weight, but sometimes dry weights are used. Animals consist on average of about 70% water, so a concentration expressed on a dry weight basis will be 3–4 times as large as the same concentration expressed on a wet weight basis. Occasionally concentrations are expressed in terms of the weight of fat, particularly for organochlorine insecticides, which will give a higher figure still. So it is important, when comparing residues, to be sure that they are all expressed in the same units. Unless stated to the contrary, one can usually assume that fresh weights are implied. Secondly, wildlife specimens are sometimes already dead when collected for analysis. This introduces two additional sources of error. Water can be lost from the corpse, when 'fresh weight' measurements will be too low, and pollutants may continue to be metabolised after death. We have already discussed the conversion of DDT to DDD, but it is a more serious problem with the organophosphorus insecticides. These are rapidly broken down, so much so that a corpse which was killed by organophosphorus insecticide poisoning may have no detectable residues when analysed. Attempts are being made to overcome this by measuring the activity of enzymes which are affected by these insecticides.

One of the first questions which must be asked in any quantitative work is, how accurate are the measurements? Given, say, a 'cleaned-up' extract of adipose tissue from an animal that contains DDE, repeated analyses of samples from the extract will not normally give identical results, or estimates. The answers will vary, with most falling relatively close to the average or mean value of all the determinations, and a few falling relatively far above or below the average. The accuracy of the mean value increases as the number of estimates increases, and, for a given number of estimates, the smaller the variation between estimates the greater the accuracy of the mean. This variation between estimates is due to various factors, the details varying with the type of analysis. For instance, in our example, the volume of extract, and therefore the amount of DDE, that is injected into the gas–liquid chromatograph will probably differ slightly from injection to injection. The accuracy of the mean can usually be indicated by the 'standard error', which, loosely speaking, is a measure of the average amount by which estimates of the mean might be expected to deviate from the true mean. Thus analysis might show that our extract of adipose tissue contained 1.63 ± 0.04 ppm DDE: here the mean is 1.63 and the standard error is 0.04. If the mean is based on a lot of estimates, there are about seven chances in ten that the actual concentration of DDE lies within the range $1.63 - 0.04$ to $1.63 + 0.04$ ppm, or within the range $1.59 - 1.67$ ppm. If the mean is based on only a few estimates, the range will be wider than the mean $\pm$ the standard error. The probabilities of other ranges about the mean can easily be calculated from the standard error. One of the most commonly used ranges is plus and minus twice the standard error. For large samples there are nineteen chances in twenty that the actual value lies within this range. It is a commonly accepted convention that the actual value does in fact fall within this range—the one chance in twenty that it will actually be outside this range is taken to be so small that it can safely be ignored—scientists take a different view of life from gamblers. This notation is standard in the scientific publication of results, and does emphasise the fact that our measurements are indeed estimates, and not absolute values.

In the example quoted the estimate is a reasonably accurate one. However, there are other types of error too.

One of the more difficult types of error to deal with is called bias. It is common knowledge amongst workers on pollution that when a tissue extract is prepared for analysis some of the insecticide is lost during the various chemical procedures. The amount lost varies with the tissue, but it is commonly within the range 10–30 % of the total for organochlorine insecticides. This loss can be estimated by adding a known, comparable, amount of the pollutant to a piece of uncontaminated tissue, treating it in exactly the same way, and comparing the estimated value with the expected value. This test does assume of course that insecticide added to a specimen will be extracted with the same efficiency as insecticide which has been incorporated into the tissue whilst the animal was alive. Obviously all estimates of residue concentrations are biased, and are too low because of the losses during extraction and 'clean-up'. Sometimes the estimates are corrected for this bias.

This bias is only significant because there are only small amounts of pollutant present—bias of this sort ceases to be a problem with higher concentrations. There is in fact a continual pressure on analytical chemists engaged in pollution research for more and yet more sensitive analytical techniques, able to detect smaller and smaller concentrations. In such a situation the accuracy of the analyses relies heavily on the skill of the analyst. Analysts tend to refer to the current stage of development of their techniques as 'the state of the art', and it must be admitted that sometimes one's confidence in the validity of an analytical result depends mainly on who did the analysis. Many laboratories do of course publish analytical results, and if these results are to be usefully compared with each other the analyses must be comparable. A comparative survey was made of seventeen laboratories, in eleven countries, a few years ago, under the auspices of OECD, to see just how comparable their analyses were for organochlorine insecticides. The personnel in these laboratories were experienced in this type of work, and the results were reassuring. There were four samples. The first was a solution of six known residues, whilst the other three were biological specimens where, by the nature of the case, the true concentrations were unknown. The estimates for the standard solution were close to the true values except for endrin, which was surprisingly low (Table 5-1). Agreement between estimates for the other three samples depended on how difficult 'clean-up' was. The results can be summarised by saying that analytical errors affected the answer by less than a factor of two, unless of course there was an undetected bias. So these results suggest that an analytical result for an organochlorine insecticide obtained by an experienced analyst should be not less than half, and not more than twice, the true value. One must emphasise the word experienced. Canadian workers have found that results from inexperienced laboratories can be far less accurate.

This covers most of the sources of error that are likely to occur with a single sample. In practice, one is also concerned with either the

Table 5–1. Estimates from seventeen laboratories for the concentrations of six organochlorine insecticide residues in a known solution. (Data from A. V. Holden, 1970.)

Compound	pp′–DDT	pp′–DDE	pp′–DDD	Dieldrin	Endrin	Heptachlor
Actual concentration (mg/litre)	9.95	4.87	10.04	5.24	7.05	4.95
Means and standard errors of estimates (mg/litre)	9.90 ±0.17	4.93 ±0.12	9.96 ±0.18	5.25 ±0.10	5.93 ±0.25	4.91 ±0.14

variation between experimental animals given identical exposures, or the variation between individual animals taken from a wild population. The amount of variation between experimental animals will depend largely on the skill of the experimenter, but with field samples it is another matter—one has, to a large extent, to take things as they are. And it is here that the really large-scale variations can occur.

The Swedes have done much of the important work on mercury as a pollutant, and they compiled a very interesting set of data on the concentrations of mercury found in the livers of pheasants (*Phasianus colchicus*). They divided the data into two groups, those from pheasants which were shot dead, and those from pheasants which were found already dead. They are summarised in Table 5-2, and show three

Table 5–2. Concentrations (ppm) of mercury found in the livers of pheasants. (Data from K. Borg, H. Wanntorp, K. Erne & E. Hanko, 1969.)

Type of sample	Number of birds	% of birds within these ranges of mercury concentration						
		0–1	1.1–2	2.1–5	5.1–10	10.1–20	20.1–40	>40
Found dead	102	49.0	18.6	15.7	10.8	2.0	1.0	2.9
Shot dead	78	59.0	16.7	15.4	6.4	2.6	—	—

salient features. There is a considerable range of values, far greater than could conceivably be ascribed to analytical error. With such a range it is likely that, if the concentrations are high enough to have any deleterious effects, some individuals will be far more affected than others. Secondly, the individual values have a skew distribution. That is to say, the distribution of individual values about the mean is asymmetric. In both groups about half of the birds contained less than 1 ppm, but there is a long 'tail' above the mean of a few relatively large values. These two characteristics, of a wide range of values that have a skew distribution, suggest that there is a risk that any sample of individuals taken from a population for analysis will be biased. And this is the third characteristic of the data in Table 5-2: if one can assume that pheasants which were shot are a random sample of all the pheasants, then the pheasants found dead give a biased estimate, for on average they contain significantly higher concentrations of mercury. A random sample is one in which all individuals have the same probability of being selected, and often the way in which samples are taken is such that those few individuals with high concentrations, which are the most affected, are either more or less likely to be included in the sample than are those with smaller amounts of pollutant. In the example of the pheasants, the individuals with very high concentrations are more likely to die than is the rest of the population. So a collection of corpses is likely to be biased in favour of birds with high concentrations.

Once one has made due allowance for these various pitfalls, and has what one considers to be a realistic picture of the residues present, what does this tell us about past exposure to the pollutant? Much of the relevant information has come from laboratory experiments, in which animals are kept in rather uniform conditions, with known constant exposures to one or more pollutants. Life in the field is of course far more variable, but it is useful first to consider relatively simple situations. In these experiments, aquatic organisms are commonly exposed to pollutants in the water, which is either frequently or continuously replaced so as to maintain a constant concentration. Terrestrial species are commonly given standard concentrations of pollutant in their food.

Imagine a fish swimming in an aquarium and exposed to a constant concentration of dieldrin in the water. The concentration is low enough to avoid any apparent adverse effects on the fish. At first the concentration of dieldrin in the fish will rise rapidly, but as the amount in the fish increases, the rate at which it increases will begin to slow down, until eventually a steady state is reached in which the amount in the body stays constant: (see diagram at top of p. 62).

One might suppose that this plateau indicated that the fish was no longer taking in any dieldrin. This is however an unlikely explanation. The continuance of life depends on the maintenance of

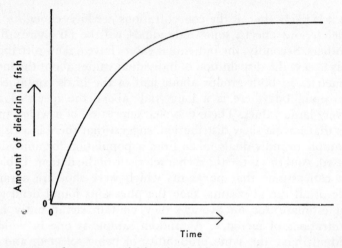

numerous steady states within the body, e.g. the concentration of glucose in blood, and these steady states are always dynamic situations, in which a fairly constant value, or steady state, is maintained because the rate at which various processes are tending to raise the concentration equals the rate at which other processes are tending to lower the concentration. So we may suppose that when our fish attains the plateau concentration for dieldrin then the rate at which dieldrin enters the body equals the sum of the rates at which it is excreted and metabolised. It follows then that if the concentration of dieldrin in the water rises or falls, there will be a corresponding change in the plateau concentration in the fish, albeit after a time-lag.

When exposure to dieldrin ceases, then the concentration of dieldrin in the fish starts to drop, and in the simplest situation there is often a simple relationship between time after end of exposure and amount in the body. A graph with normal arithmetic scales along the axes shows a smooth curve:

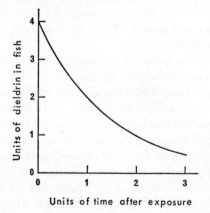

The shape of the curve is such that the percentage drop after any given interval of time is constant. If, for example, the concentration dropped from 20 to 10 ppm in two weeks, then after a further two weeks the concentration would have dropped to 5 ppm. This is precisely the same pattern as occurs with the rate of decay of radioactive isotopes. It is standard practice to measure the rate of decay for such isotopes in terms of their half-lives, i.e. that interval of time in which the radioactivity has decreased by half. It is not strictly correct to refer to the half-life of a pollutant in an organism, because, unlike radioactivity, the rate of loss of a pollutant is likely to be affected by environmental changes, and also there are deviations from the expected values. Such curves can easily be converted to straight lines by using a geometric scale on the vertical axis of the graph:

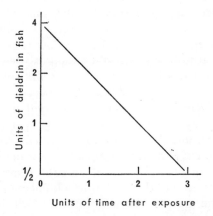

Units of time after exposure

Experimentally, straight lines are much to be preferred. It is much easier to fit a straight line to a set of experimental values than it is to fit a curve. It is also much easier to summarise all the relevant information for a straight line than a curve. The angle that the line makes to the horizontal tells one how persistent the pollutant is within the organism: the steeper the line, the more rapidly the pollutant is lost. This may seem platitudinous, but it does allow us to express in precise quantitative terms, with standard errors, the relative persistence of different compounds, or of the same compound in different species or in different environmental situations. In practice, although there have been many experimental studies of this sort, the data have rarely been expressed in this form, so that such comparisons are almost impossible to make. However, it should be possible to extract information on rates of intake and loss from the published data. One might hope that then in time we will have

E

information for each pollutant of its likely rates of intake by, and of persistence within, organisms.

It is true that the experimental results for loss of residues from specific tissues or organs within the body do often fall onto straight lines of this type. There are theoretical reasons though, supported by some of the more extensive sets of experimental data, for supposing that loss of residues after exposure follows a more complicated pattern. The percentage drop per unit of time, or rate of loss, is not constant, but tends to decrease with time. This decrease in the rate of loss has not been shown very often, in part perhaps because research workers were not looking out for it, and tend to assume that residues are lost at a constant rate. In addition, this decreased rate of loss sometimes becomes apparent only after a long time, of some months, and many experiments do not last that long. Either way, the fact of a decreasing rate of loss with increasing time after exposure has one interesting consequence. Some pollutants, such as DDE, appear to be virtually ubiquitous in wildlife samples. It is sometimes deduced that such pollutants must occur, in very low concentrations, everywhere. This is possibly correct—the amounts present would be too small to be detected without the greatest difficulty. But it is also conceivable that organisms far from the sources of pollutants have occasional relatively high exposures, and that a small part of the residues acquired at such times is exceedingly persistent.

There is another useful relationship between exposure and residues. The concentration of pesticide within an organism obviously depends on the exposure. In general terms, the greater the exposure, either as a higher concentration in the food or as a higher concentration in the environment, the greater the concentration within the organism. There is often in fact a fairly simple relationship between the two (Fig. 5-1).

The field situation is of course far more complex. Exposure is likely to be inconstant, and other conditions too, which may affect the relationship between exposure and residues, may fluctuate. However, these inconstancies do not always cause too violent deviations from the neat experimental results. A four-acre marsh on the shore of Lake Erie, USA, was sprayed from the air in 1964 with DDT, in granular form, at 0.2 lb/acre. Plant, animal, water and mud samples were taken at intervals and analysed for residues. The DDT was labelled with radioactive chlorine, which was attached to the phenyl groups in the normal *para para* positions. Samples were analysed for radioactivity. Strictly this measurement only tells one how much radioactive chlorine is present. In practice it is probably a good measure for the total quantity of DDT plus metabolites that is present in the sample, but it is impossible by this method to

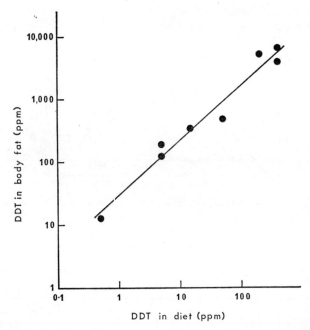

Fig. 5-1 Concentrations of DDT in the fat of female rats fed DDT in their diet for up to six months. (Data from W. J. Hayes, 1959.)

distinguish DDT from the rest. A selection of the results is shown in Fig. 5-2.

The concentration in the water, from which the particulate matter had been removed, rose rapidly, and within twelve hours after spraying had reached about the theoretical maximum solubility of DDT in water, although, as discussed in chapter two, this is a somewhat hypothetical value. All radioactivity had disappeared from the water within one month of spraying. Suspended particulate matter in the water ceased to have any detectable radioactivity within the first week, but the surface sediments of the marsh remained remarkably constant, at about 0.3 ppm, from the time that the first sample was taken, six weeks after spraying, until at least fifteen months after spraying. R. L. Meeks analysed many plant and animal species, and the typical pattern was that they attained maximal values within a week, and had much higher concentrations than the water. The plateau value for most animal species was of the order of 1–10 ppm, which was 1,000–10,000 times higher than the concentrations in water, from which presumably the organisms acquired their DDT. These data illustrate very clearly the remarkable facility that living organisms possess for concentrating organochlorine insecticides from the physical environment. However, it is also noteworthy that

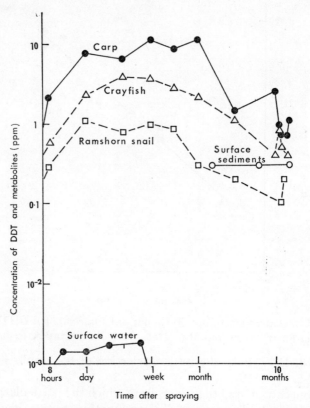

Fig. 5-2. The concentration of DDT plus metabolites in samples taken from a 4-acre marsh sprayed with 0.2 lb DDT/acre. (Data taken from R. L. Meeks, 1968.)

although the highest concentrations occur within organisms, the residues found in the surface sediments suggest that most of the DDT sprayed onto the marsh became 'locked-up' in this part of the physical environment, just because the mass of sediments was presumably much larger than the biomass. With results like these it is no longer so surprising to find that these compounds are so widespread in wildlife. The plants and animals then started to lose their DDT after the first week or so, when their exposure to DDT in the water virtually ceased. It is noteworthy that the residues were lost far more slowly than they were acquired.

This is not always the pattern. Some other American workers studied the persistence of DDT in coniferous forests in Maine that had been sprayed once with DDT at 1 lb/acre. The concentration of DDT in the soil remained steady at about 1 ppm for at least nine years after spraying. Not surprisingly, they found too that earthworms (various species) and robins (*Turdus migratorius*) from these forests had fairly constant concentrations of both DDT and of metabolites. This does not necessarily indicate that the DDT persists indefinitely in the soil. It could be that the DDT in the soil is continually replenished by the insecticide coming into the soil from the trees above. Whatever the explanation, it is clear that the population of robins and of earthworms in this situation maintain a plateau level of residues for many years.

It is obvious from these two sets of results that analysis of a few specimens from a population at one time gives relatively little information on exposure. One will not know whether the population has reached a plateau concentration, or whether residues are on the increase or decrease. They are often useful though in deciding whether observed deaths are due to pollutants and, at sublethal levels, they can indicate, for that particular time, whether the population is near to or far from acutely toxic levels.

We must delve a little more deeply before we can assess the relevance of residue levels for predicting the potential risk of acute toxicity. It is common with vertebrates to analyse specific tissues for pollutants. Birds' eggs and invertebrates are commonly analysed whole, but a peregrine falcon say would present an inconveniently large sample to prepare for analysis. It is much simpler to dissect out small quantities from specific tissues. The same relationships between exposure and concentration apply to tissues as to whole organisms. It is also found that, given a stable situation where all relevant factors remain constant, the concentrations in different tissues are in constant proportions to each other. The highest concentrations of organochlorine insecticides occur in adipose tissue. It is well established that if the fat reserves are mobilised by starvation, then some of the residues will be released from the adipose tissue, and concentrations will rise in other tissues. If the concentration in the fat is high enough, and the starvation is severe enough, then sufficient insecticide may be released to other tissues for the animal to die. This process is important when predicting the risk of acute toxicity.

An interesting experiment by D. J. Jefferies and B. N. K. Davis at Monks Wood illustrates this point. They fed five song thrushes (*Turdus ericetorum*) on earthworms (*Lumbricus terrestris*) for six weeks. Some of the earthworms contained dieldrin, and each bird was given a different daily dose of dieldrin. The bird on the top dose died after only nine days. None of the other four birds showed any symptoms of dieldrin poisoning during six weeks exposure. They were then killed and analysed for residues. Extrapolation from the residues in the four unaffected birds suggested that the bird on the top dose should, if it had survived for the whole six weeks, have had 3.1 ppm dieldrin in its brain. In fact, although it had only lived for the first nine days of the experiment it had more than five times this concentration, with 16.9 ppm dieldrin in its brain. We do not know whether or not the birds had all reached their plateau concentrations before they were analysed. If not, the difference between the actual and predicted value for the bird on the top dose is even greater than the figures suggest. Jefferies and Davis suggested that this unexpectedly high concentration happened because the bird mobilised much of its fat reserves before death, thus releasing much dieldrin into the blood and raising the concentration of dieldrin in the brain: the bird had used up all its storage fat before it died. In fact, it is commonly found that animals which have died from insecticide poisoning have reduced fat reserves. This reduction probably has at least two causes. Animals may stop eating during the early symptoms of poisoning. There is also evidence to suggest that food reserves are used up faster than would be expected during normal starvation. The inference is that the hyperactive stage of poisoning must use up a considerable amount of energy.

The practical significance of these results is as follows. We know that the primary lesion that causes death occurs in the nervous system, and experiments show, as might be expected, that the probability of death from insecticide poisoning depends on the concentration of insecticide in the brain. It is found, as a very rough guide, that concentrations of dieldrin above 5 ppm in dead birds suggest strongly that dieldrin was the cause of death. There are assumptions of course. Often one has to assume that results from one species are applicable to another, and one ignores the possible effects of third variables—how does a small amount of another pollutant, or a physiological stress such as inclement weather, affect the animal's response? If then one assumes 5 ppm in the brain to be the critical level at which death is likely to occur, and one finds a wild population has about 1 ppm in the brain, one might argue, assuming the population to have reached a plateau level, that the exposure is such that the brain concentration would have to be five times as great to reach the critical level. In fact, the thrush results suggest that such a population is in imminent danger, for once the symptoms of poisoning start the amount of dieldrin in the brain will rise sharply.

These data also showed some other interesting features (Table 5-3). The concentration in the thrushes was lower than that in their diet, although if the thrushes had not yet reached their plateau levels they might eventually have exceeded it. Perhaps of greater significance is the low proportion of the ingested insecticide that is retained within the body. In this example, it was less than 5% for all diets,

Table 5-3. The retention and concentration of dieldrin in four song thrushes (*Turdus ericetorum*) fed contaminated earthworms for six weeks. All concentrations are based on wet weights. (Data from D. J. Jefferies & B. N. K. Davis, 1968.)

Bird	Concentration of dieldrin in diet (ppm)	Total amount of dieldrin eaten with the earthworms (micrograms)	Total amount of dieldrin in body after 6 weeks (micrograms)	% of dieldrin in diet present in body	Concentration of dieldrin in body (ppm)	Concentration in body as % of that in diet
A	0.15	203.6	1.54	0.8	0.02	13.3
B	0.32	436.8	7.11	1.6	0.09	28.1
C	3.06	3837.0	96.0	2.5	1.36	44.4
D	5.69	7297.0	318.0	4.4	4.03	70.8

and for the lowest dose rate was less than 1 %. One could of course deduce this second feature from the asymptotic nature of the increase in body concentration with time. When a plateau concentration has been reached, there is still a continued ingestion of insecticide, but the amount present in the body remains constant. Thus the longer the period of exposure, the lower becomes the percentage of the dose that is retained.

This conclusion runs starkly counter to the conventional wisdom about the persistent organochlorine insecticides, which was first disseminated amongst the lay public by Rachel Carson in her book *Silent Spring*, published in 1962. She concluded that animals in successive links of a food chain contain higher concentrations of residues than do their prey species. She then stated that these higher concentrations in predators are obtained by storing the accumulations from their prey species. This idea has become widely accepted, including many of those involved professionally with these problems. Much of the evidence shows this generalisation to be false, but the subject provides some startling examples of the power of myth over fact— whatever the logical deductions from a set of facts may be, they are sometimes adduced as evidence for accumulation of persistent pesticides along food chains, even when they suggest the opposite.

The idea of food chains is virtually self-explanatory. It was first put formally by C. Elton, in 1927. All animals are selective in what they eat, but all depend, directly or indirectly, on plants for their energy. Plant feeders form the first link in the chain, and these are usually preyed on by carnivores, which may themselves be preyed on by other species, till eventually we reach a species, such as the peregrine falcon, which has no predators. Most food chains are quite short, consisting of only two or three species, and it is more usual nowadays to think of the feeding relationships between species as forming a food web, rather than food chains. Predators are rarely specific feeders on only one species, and if one species is scarce or absent then the predator will feed on another species.

Carson's conclusions were based on some events at Clear Lake, California. This is an irregularly shaped lake, about nineteen miles long and seven miles wide, in the mountains ninety miles north of San Francisco. Clear Lake is important for recreation—fishing, picnicking and so forth. Unfortunately large numbers of the gnat *Chaoborus astictopus* breed in this lake, and the adults were so numerous that they were a severe nuisance to visitors. Because of this nuisance, the lake was sprayed with DDD in 1949. The spraying was done from barges, and the amount used was such that if it were dispersed uniformly throughout the water in the body of the lake the estimated concentration was 0.014 ppm. This is, as we discussed in chapter two, an unrealistic assumption, but there were no measurements of the actual distribution of insecticide. Control of the gnat was virtually complete, but by 1954 the lake had to be sprayed again, and it was sprayed a third time three years later, in 1957. On both these later occasions the theoretical concentration of DDD in the water was 0.02 ppm. One of the attractive wildlife features of the lake was the number of western grebes (*Aechmophorus occidentalis*); about 100 dead specimens of this bird were found about three months after the application of both the second and third sprays. E. G. Hunt and A. I. Bischoff investigated the reasons for these deaths, and concluded that probably the birds had died from DDD poisoning—they had 1,600 ppm of DDD in their fatty tissue. There is no reason to doubt this explanation, but the occurrence of such high concentrations of DDD was remarkable, when judged by the knowledge available at that time. This DDD was thought to have come via the grebes' food, fish. Analyses of fish taken at various times during the year after the third application showed that they attained even higher concentrations of DDD in their visceral fat, up to 2,690 ppm. There was no evidence for sudden unexpected deaths of fish, so Hunt and Bischoff suggested that the grebes were more susceptible to the DDD than many of the species of fish in the lake. They then went on to make some rather more debatable suggestions. They said that carnivorous fish had higher concentrations of DDD than did plankton-eating fish, and that this difference was a result of their different positions in the food chain. Many of their samples of fish were taken at different times, so that the exposures to DDD were different, but if one assumes either that this makes no difference, or that the effects of different exposures applied equally to all age groups, then the data

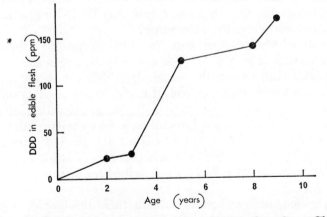

Fig. 5-3. Concentrations of DDD in white catfish taken from Clear Lake in October, 1958. (Data taken from E. G. Hunt & A. I. Bischoff, 1960.)

suggest strongly that the older fish have higher concentrations (e.g. Fig. 5-3). Admittedly there is a very wide scatter in the values for individual specimens within some of the age groups, but the results do show one relevant conclusion very clearly. Comparisons between species of fish should be with fish of similar ages. More recent work has shown that older fish often do have higher concentrations of organochlorine insecticides, although the exact reasons are not too clearly understood at present.

When one excludes comparisons between fish of different ages, there is only one valid comparison available from Hunt and Bischoff's results. This was for analyses of muscle from a plankton-eating fish and a carnivorous fish (Table 5-4). It is true that the carnivore had

Table 5-4. Analyses of muscle from composite samples of two species of fish taken from Clear Lake, California. (Data from E. G. Hunt & A. I. Bischoff, 1960.)

Species	Feeding habits	Concentration of DDD (ppm)	Concentration of fat (%)
Sacramento blackfish (*Orthodon microlepidotus*)	Plankton eater	7–9	1.5
Largemouth bass (*Micropterus salmoides*)	Carnivore	22–25	6.0

about three times as high a concentration of DDD in its muscle as the plankton eater, but it is also true that the carnivore's muscle had four times as much fat in it as the plankton eater's. So one could argue that like is not being compared with like. There are at least two possible explanations: the carnivorous fish has more DDD in its muscle either because of its position in the food chain, or because its muscle has more fat in it. The latter appears to be quite a reasonable explanation, because we know that DDD is fat-soluble, and because fatty tissues do have the highest concentrations of DDD. Hunt and Bischoff's suggestion does imply of course that DDD is absorbed via the food, and not direct from the water.

The results of Meeks' experiment, in which he sprayed a four-acre marsh with DDT (Fig. 5-2), suggest that aquatic organisms take in the insecticide direct from the water. It is difficult to see how, if DDT were obtained from the food, it could have passed so quickly along the food chain to the carp. All species, regardless of their position in the food chain, appeared to have very similar patterns for accumulation of DDT. In fairness to Hunt and Bischoff it must be added that this is the wisdom of hindsight. Meeks' work, and other relevant work, came after they had described the situation at Clear Lake.

This question, of whether fish obtain their residues of organochlorine insecticides direct from the water, or via the food, is very easy to test experimentally. R. E. Reinert was the first person to describe a critical test. He chose three species, a fish, crustacean and alga, which could form a simple experimental food chain. These three species, the common guppy (*Lebistes reticulatus*), *Daphnia magna* and the alga *Scenedesmus obliquus*, were kept in separate aquaria with fairly constant concentrations of dieldrin. The only possible source of dieldrin was from the water. Specimens were analysed at intervals until they had reached plateau concentrations. Even though all three species could only have obtained their dieldrin from the water, the size of the dieldrin residues was correlated with each species position in the food chain:

Species	*Concentration factor* (i.e. plateau concentration of dieldrin in dried animals, divided by the concentration of dieldrin in the water)
Alga	1,282
Daphnia	13,954
Guppy	49,307

In other experiments, guppies were fed contaminated *Daphnia*, and there was no significant rise in the fishes' dieldrin residues. A similar result was obtained for *Daphnia* that fed on contaminated algae. In fact, direct intake from the water is a sufficient explanation for the increase in concentration up the food chain. In other words, the fact that the higher members of this food chain have the higher concentrations of dieldrin is coincidental, and is not because the dieldrin accumulates and concentrates up the food chain.

This conclusion was confirmed in another series of experiments by G. G. Chadwick and R. W. Brocksen, who exposed another fish species, the reticulate sculpin (*Cottus perplexus*), to a concentration of 0.5×10^{-3} ppm HEOD for up to 21 days. The fish were fed on worms. One group of fish was fed with worms which had been given the same exposure to HEOD as the fish. Both groups of fish had reached virtually plateau concentrations of HEOD in their bodies by the end of three weeks, and they contained similar amounts of HEOD. Obviously the amount of HEOD in the fish was not influenced by the presence or absence of HEOD in the fishes' food. This result was reinforced by the fact that, by the end of the three weeks, only 16% of the total amount of HEOD in the fish could have come from the contaminated worms. Doubtless some of the HEOD from the worms was eliminated by the fish, thus reducing still further the food's contribution to the total residues in the fish.

It is important to add one qualification. It could be that some species within a habitat have a greater exposure than other species, because of their different behaviour. It is conceivable that then food would be an important source of organochlorine insecticides for predators. We have little information on the likelihood of this arising in practice.

From these and other observations and experiments one can conclude that, for aquatic organisms, position in the food chain is not directly relevant to the amount of insecticide that is accumulated. It remains of course an interesting question to ask why fish often have higher concentrations of these pollutants than do aquatic invertebrates, but it is important that we dismiss the notion that concentration up the food chain is the answer. Until we set this idea aside we will never be able to ask the right questions.

Before we consider terrestrial food chains, there is one other detail about Clear Lake, as described by Rachel Carson, which must be corrected. She said that 'plankton organisms were found to contain about 5 parts per million of the insecticide'. In fact Hunt and Bischoff state unequivocally in their paper that they could not detect any DDD in the plankton, probably because the sample was too small, although they did find 10.9 ppm of DDD in a plankton sample taken a year later.

So one of the principal conclusions to be drawn from Clear Lake is, as with the pregrine falcon, that animals have a high affinity for organochlorine insecticides.

Terrestrial species do presumably, outside of sprayed areas, obtain their insecticide from their food. There is some evidence, from analyses of field specimens, to suggest that the amount of insecticide which terrestrial species contain does depend on their position in the food chain. N. W. Moore and C. H. Walker published results of a preliminary survey they made of British birds to get some idea of the amounts present in a wide range of species. There were of course considerable differences between individual specimens of each species, but overall there was quite a marked correlation between type of food and size of residue. They found that breast muscle from predatory birds had higher concentrations of organochlorine insecticide residues than that from herbivorous birds, whilst insectivores had an intermediate position (Fig. 5-4). Other workers have since published similar results. Should we therefore conclude that for species which obtain persistent pollutants from their food, and not direct from the physical environment, there is an increase in concentration up the food chain?

Some facts must be established, or assumptions made, before we can safely make this deduction from such residue data. If we can suppose that our estimates of how much pollutant occurs in animals are unbiased for each species, and that each species has reached a steady state, with a more or less constant amount of pollutant, then data such as those of Moore and Walker show clearly that predators

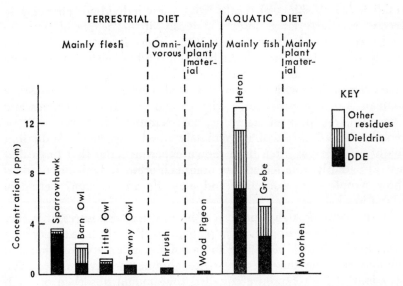

Fig. 5-4. Amounts of organochlorine insecticides found in breast muscle of birds (after N. W. Moore & C. H. Walker, 1964).

have higher concentrations of organochlorine insecticides than do herbivores. This could be because of their relative positions in the food chain, with predators having a higher exposure to insecticides from their food than do the herbivores. Alternatively, it could be because predators tend to accumulate more from a given exposure—they might, for example, tend to be less able to metabolise insecticides. However, we do not know at present whether these initial assumptions, of unbiased estimates and steady states, are correct. We only have a few suggestive facts and ideas.

In the first place, it seems unlikely that terrestrial species ever do experience anything like a constant exposure to pollutants. Agricultural applications of pesticides are of course very intermittent, and one has no good reason to suppose that the rate of release into the environment is constant for other pollutants. Moreover, the amounts of pollutants vary from place to place, so that a mobile animal will experience varying exposures not only because of fluctuations with time in the amounts present, but also as a result of its movements. We do not know what pattern of residue concentrations would occur with irregular exposures, but this could well be the usual mode of exposures. We have already seen that the decline in the population of peregrine falcons was attributed to acute toxicity after a sudden large intake of dieldrin. Deaths of some badgers and foxes have also been explained by similar patterns of poisoning with insecticides. It has also been suggested that the skew distribution commonly found with residues (e.g. Table 5-2) results from a few individuals chancing to receive relatively large doses. Obviously, if the degree of exposure varies considerably from time to time, there is no possibility of a steady state being reached. At best the residue levels will fluctuate about a stable mean, and will resemble somewhat the temperature chart of a patient with high fever. It is also debatable how realistic a plateau level is anyway for a wild animal. Survival is arduous and uncertain. At times of starvation for example fat reserves will be mobilised, and this will immediately upset any steady state that might exist. It has often been shown experimentally that birds that are apparently unaffected by organochlorine insecticide residues show symptoms of poisoning and may die after a short period of starvation.

If one assumes such a pattern of intermittent exposures, it is easy to envisage that attainment of a 'plateau level' might take a very long time. Such a level would have to be defined as a situation where, in the long run, the amount of pesticide eliminated between successive occasions of high exposure equalled the amount absorbed on such occasions. Such a stage could conceivably take several years to attain. Predators tend in general to be longer lived than their prey, and their greater longevity could then be an adequate explanation for their higher residues. Unfortunately I do not know of any adequate data to test this idea on the size of residues found in terrestrial predators of different ages.

Another possible explanation for higher residue levels in terrestrial predators would be that they select out the most heavily contaminated of their prey species. Predators do often ensure the fitness of their prey species by preying on the ailing individuals. Similarly one might expect that individual prey affected by a pollutant may be selected by predators. A colleague and I once tried to test this idea, by putting a house sparrow in a room with a few dosed and undosed butterflies. Eventually we abandoned the project: either the bird was not interested because it was full up, or we could not manage to prevent its eating all of the butterflies before we had a chance to identify the survivors. However, Cooke contrived a more satisfactory experimental situation. He placed single warty newts (*Triturus cristatus*) in an aquarium, and introduced pairs of frog tadpoles (*Rana temporaria*). One of each pair was normal, the other was hyperactive from DDT poisoning. If it were a matter of indifference to the newt whether or not tadpoles were affected by DDT, one would expect that, on average, it would eat the dosed tadpole first in half of the total number of trials. In fact the dosed tadpole was eaten first in ninety trials out of one hundred. This is a far greater deviation from a 50:50 ratio than could be expected by chance, so the inference is that, in that situation, newts eat hyperactive tadpoles in preference to normal ones. No shelter was provided in the aquarium. It would be interesting to see whether the same result was obtained in an aquarium with plenty of cover.

Of course, if selection of the most heavily contaminated prey is the reason for higher levels in predators, it is still true that position in the food chain does affect the amount of residue. The same applies to one of the other suggestions, that predators as a group are less efficient than herbivores at disposing of foreign compounds. But it does mean, as with aquatic food chains, that the emphasis should be transferred from position in food chain to rates of intake and elimination. Certainly two points do deserve emphasis. All living organisms appear to have a great facility for acquiring persistent insecticides from the physical environment, and much if not most of the insecticide that is acquired is subsequently eliminated—the higher concentrations that remain are only a fraction of those that have been taken into the body.

To conclude these surmises, it can be shown that if species A is eaten by species B, that individuals of species B feed only on species A, and that individuals of both species have steady state concentrations of pollutant, then,

$$\frac{\text{concentration of pollutant in B}}{\text{concentration of pollutant in A}} = \frac{\text{daily food intake by B as \% of body weight}}{\text{daily loss of residues from B as \% of total residues}}$$

To express it simply, given a few assumptions, a predator will tend to have higher concentrations of pollutant than its prey if its food intake exceeds its rate of excretion and metabolism. We have very few data on either food intake by wild animals or the rate at which they lose residues. However, this relationship shows clearly that the more slowly a species loses its residues, the more likely it is to have higher residues than its prey. In the extreme case of course, where no loss occurs, one would indeed have the situation where residues would concentrate and accumulate along the food chain.

The idea that persistent pollutants may concentrate and accumulate along food chains has aroused great public interest. In part, this interest is probably self-centred. Our own species is at the end of many food chains, with the implication that we are particularly at risk from such compounds. The data from autopsies in the United Kingdom are reassuring: the amounts of organochlorine insecticides in the body fat of our own species have declined since the mid-1960s. This is what we might expect. Our exposure to organochlorine insecticides probably reached a peak in the 1960s, and our residues have declined as the degree of exposure has declined. Implicit in this commonsense explanation is the idea of a steady state, which we have already discussed. Most of the experimental evidence supports the idea that, with chronic exposure, the rate of loss eventually equals the rate of intake, and the idea has been extensively tested in similar studies with drugs. It must be admitted however that the experimental evidence for DDT and dieldrin in our own species does not suggest that a steady state is reached.

In an experiment with volunteers amongst convicts in the USA, adult males ingested DDT for 21.5 months. Four dose rates were used. There were occasional mistakes, with an individual receiving the wrong dose, and it is therefore only worthwhile to consider the results for those men receiving the largest doses, of 35 mg technical grade or 35 mg recrystallised DDT/day. An occasional missed dose should not have had much effect on their residues. Fat samples from the volunteers were taken before dosing started, and 12.2, 18.8 and 21.5 months later. The results with both technical grade and pure DDT suggest a steady rise with time in the amounts of DDT stored in the fat (Fig. 5-5).

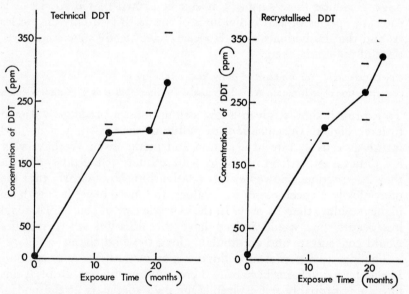

Fig. 5-5. Amounts of DDT in the body fat of adult men whilst ingesting 35 mg DDT (technical grade or recrystallised)/day. Standard errors are indicated by the horizontal bars. (Original data by W. J. Hayes, W. E. Dale & C. I. Pirkle, 1971.)

A similar experiment was carried out at Shell's research laboratories at Sittingbourne in England. Adult male volunteers ingested 50 or 211 microgrammes of dieldrin each day for two years. Blood samples were analysed at frequent intervals. Again, after an initial relatively rapid rise in blood levels, the concentrations in the blood rose steadily for the entire two years (Fig. 5-6).

I must state that the interpretations of these results are my own. The original authors concluded, in both instances, from statistical tests, that a steady state concentration was reached within about 18 months. The details of the statistical tests, which were quite sophisticated for the dieldrin data, need not concern us now—I am content to let the raw data speak for themselves. I do not accept the aphorism

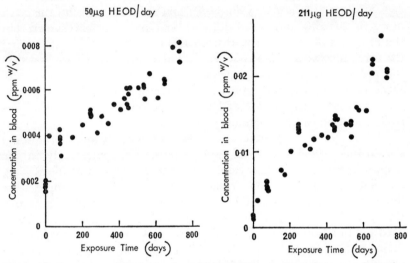

Fig. 5-6. Amounts of dieldrin found in the blood of adult men whilst ingesting 50 or 211 μg dieldrin/day. Each point represents the mean value for samples taken from three men. (Original data by C. G. Hunter, J. Robinson & M. Roberts, 1969.)

that there are lies, damned lies, and statistics. In fact statistical tests can, in suitable circumstances, provide a very powerful means of obtaining information and testing ideas. It is simply that in these two instances, in my opinion, false assumptions were made.

It seems to me to be most improbable that, in our own species, residues of organochlorine insecticides do increase indefinitely with a constant exposure. But these two studies do pose some important questions which deserve investigation.

These last sections have been speculative, and I must end this chapter by discussing one more speculation. Many thousands of tons of DDT have been used since the Second World War, and various theories have been produced to predict, both for current and other possible patterns of use, the likely future size of DDT residues in animals, especially man. Various mathematical models have been derived from these theories, and the available data used to calculate future trends. One of the more startling predictions has been that, even if we stopped all uses of DDT from tomorrow, the amounts of DDT in the higher members of food chains would continue to rise for some years yet. This seems to me to be unrealistic. I have already described the field observations on coniferous forests in Maine, where the concentration of DDT in the upper layers of the soil remained fairly constant for nine years after spraying. Likewise the residues in earthworms and robins remained fairly constant. Observations on eggs of shags (*Phalacrocorax aristotelis*) taken from islands off the coast of north-east England and south-east Scotland have also shown that the amounts of DDE, derived from DDT, tended to decline during the three successive years 1969–1971. These observations suggest that the predictions of rising levels can only be true if the amounts of DDT in some parts of the physical environment rise appreciably for some time after the release of DDT has stopped. This is not impossible, but I know of no evidence for it.

This exercise is relevant to at least one activity of international significance. DDT has been, and still is, used extensively in the tropics for the control of several important insect vectors of diseases, especially malaria. At one time about 1,800 million people were living in malarious areas. Extensive use of DDT, at one time 60,000 tons/year, has more than halved this number. The amount of DDT used for this programme of eradication and control is also down to about half of the maximum use. DDT has many advantages—it is effective, it is cheap, it has low toxicity to man, and because it is persistent it does not have to be used very often. And application is itself expensive. It has been argued that DDT should be replaced by some of the organophosphorus insecticides, so as to reduce the degree of environmental pollution. These alternatives are effective, sometimes, but they cost more, and have to be applied more frequently. This is a classic example of a conflict of interests between the 'developed' and 'under-developed' countries. A poor person who has the choice of using DDT and avoiding malaria, or of not adding to the amount of DDT in the world and having malaria, must be suicidally inclined if he doesn't use DDT. This is an over-simplified picture, but one can argue that if the 'developed' countries would prefer DDT not to be used they must be prepared to pay the extra cost. Here we have a conflict of interests, which, like many other questions about pollution, does start raising ethical and political problems.

6

'Where Have All the Butterflies Gone?'

One of my favourite pieces of imaginative writing was produced in all seriousness by a professor in biology and published in 1967, in one of the British 'quality' newspapers, 'Who knows that the crime wave and moral deterioration which is said to be affecting Britain and the world at the present time is not, in fact, the direct result of the widespread use of insecticides, and indeed of other biologically active agents, used in connection with food production and storage, . . .' He then returned to his main theme, 'If we have lost our butterflies, let us at least learn a lesson from that loss, and quickly examine the situation more closely'. The fanciful embellishments did adorn a real question which was being asked in the early 1960s. Many people had become aware of the possible harm that pesticides might cause to wildlife. There was also a widespread feeling that the numbers of British butterflies had declined considerably since before the Second World War. It was almost inevitable therefore, given the then current climate of opinion, that pesticides were said to have reduced the numbers of butterflies.

At first glance, the situation may seem somewhat analogous to that which developed with the peregrine falcon. The central question is clearly similar: what effect have pesticides had on the population sizes of British butterflies? But the differences in biology and background information imposed a completely different approach to this problem. The numbers of butterflies vary greatly from year to year, in response to environmental changes, and are not at all like the steady numbers of peregrine. In the same way that wine connoisseurs talk of vintage years, so butterfly collectors talk of good butterfly years. It follows then that any change in population size that pesticides may cause will be much less easy to detect, because of the large fluctuations that already occur. There is, in engineers' terms, a high 'noise' level. This difficulty is compounded by the fact that we have virtually no reliable data on past population sizes. Most of the information is anecdotal, of the type 'When I was a lad, there were swarms of butterflies in that field. Now there is hardly a one'. Such statements may be quite true, but they are difficult to express in numerical terms, and there is no easy way of testing their reliability. The human memory is notoriously unreliable for factual details.

Like much of the work on the peregrine falcon, this problem too was studied at Monks Wood. The approach was deceptively simple: we would take a species which was easy to breed in the laboratory, dose it with insecticide, see what sublethal effects were produced, measure how much insecticide was needed to produce these effects, and then compare these amounts with those found in field specimens. We should then be able to assess how much risk our butterflies ran from insecticides. This approach does involve various assumptions, which we shall discuss later.

First, we had to choose a species. This was simple. We wanted a common species that was indigenous to this country, and preferably not totally reliant on continental immigrants. Then we could avoid arguments about whether the putative decline was due to factors in this country or abroad. We also thought that one whose caterpillars were gregarious should withstand the high densities in which they would be bred more readily. In the event we used the small tortoise-shell (*Aglais urticae*), one of our most common native butterflies. This nymphalid butterfly has two generations each year, and the adults of the second brood, which survive over-winter in nooks and crannies, lay their eggs the following Spring. Eggs are laid in clumps on the leaves of the common stinging nettle (*Urtica dioica*), and the caterpillars which hatch from these eggs stay together as they feed on the nettle leaves, moult four times as they grow, until the fifth instar caterpillars finally wander off, spin their coccoons and pupate. The life-cycle is completed when the adult emerges from this pupa (chrysalis).

Caterpillars were dosed by putting known amounts of pure p,p'-DDT or HEOD in solution onto the surface cuticle of fifth instar caterpillars. Further development of the caterpillars, pupae and adults was then to be assessed by a few simple measurements, but we had first to measure the lethal dose. Individuals vary in the minimum amount required to kill them, and so it is relatively difficult to determine the lethal dose. In fact it took some time for early toxicologists to devise a satisfactory measurement.

Many early measurements of the toxicity of substances were made by giving a range of doses to groups of animals, and finding the largest dose that would not kill any individuals, or the smallest dose that would kill all individuals. These measures were not very satisfactory, because individuals differ in their tolerance of poisons. So if one test group had by chance a very susceptible individual, the minimum lethal dose would be very small, and if one group had a very resistant individual, the dose required to kill all of a group might be very high. Results were therefore rather inconsistent. These difficulties were overcome by measuring that dose which killed 50% of the group. A graph of the percentage kill against size of dose usually produces an S-shaped, or sigmoid, curve:

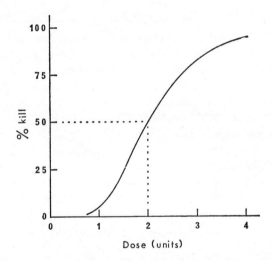

One obvious consequence of this approach is that the number of individuals in each group no longer affects the answer, except to influence the accuracy.

One can fit the best curve to the experimental values, and read off that dose which kills half of the individuals. This is commonly known as the LD_{50} (i.e. the dose that is lethal to 50% of the individuals). One can similarly measure any other dose, e.g. LD_{10}. In practice, the data are transformed to fall about a straight line. The doses are expressed on a geometric scale. Thus the difference between a dose of 2 units and one of 4 units is, in proportion, the same as the difference between a dose of 4 units and one of 8 units. The percentage kill is converted to a more complicated scale, called probits, which is readily available in books of mathematical tables. One then obtains a straight line:

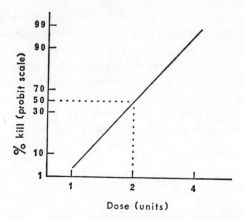

Dose (units)

The LD_{50}, with standard error, is then easily calculated.

Such experimental tests of toxicity are one form of bioassay, which have had, and still have, many uses. Essentially, one is estimating the percentage of individuals that gives a standard response to each of a range of doses of a compound. We have used death as the response, but other responses could be treated in exactly the same way, when one might measure the ED_{50} (dose that is effective in 50% of the individuals). The amounts of many biologically active compounds, such as drugs, hormones, insecticides and herbicides, can be measured by bioassay, and sometimes have to be, because chemical analytical methods either do not exist, or are too insensitive. Some at least of these bioassays can give very precise and repeatable answers, provided that standardised testing conditions are used.

In part perhaps because of this precision, LD_{50} values became something of a sacred cow in assessments of toxicity. One snag is that the answer depends so very much on the experimental conditions. J. R. Busvine gave a striking illustration in measurements of insect resistance. Many insect pests have strains which are more resistant to insecticides than are the normal susceptible individuals. The degree of resistance can be measured by comparing the LD_{50} of the resistant and of a standard susceptible strain. Busvine showed that by using two different solvents for applying DDT to houseflies the resistant strain could be shown to be either 16 or 300 times as resistant to DDT as the susceptible strain:

Solvent	LD_{50} of DDT ($\mu g/fly$)		Ratio of resistant/susceptible
	Susceptible	*Resistant*	
Mineral oil	0.44	7.2	15
Acetone	0.12	36	300

Presumably the solvent altered the amount of the applied insecticide which could penetrate the insect's cuticle and so, potentially, reach the site of action.

Temperature too can affect the response greatly. DDT is renowned for the way in which its effects are influenced by temperature, and I have had grasshoppers (*Chorthippus brunneus*) dosed with DDT, which were hyperactive and unco-ordinated at 20°C, but every time I transferred them to 25°C, their behaviour appeared perfectly normal, and conversely, when I returned them to 20°C they behaved abnormally again.

One could also expect the LD_{50} to change as an insect grows. Apart from any physiological changes, as the insect increases in weight so there is more tissue for the insecticide to be distributed in. In fact with small tortoiseshell caterpillars the situation was more complex than this, and at least two other factors were involved in the change of toxicity with growth.

The caterpillars can grow rapidly. In our experimental conditions, with ample food available, fifth instar larvae could double their weight in twenty-four hours. Weight was an accurate index of stage of development. So LD_{50} determinations were made on larvae within the weight range 80–260 mg, at intervals of 20 mg. The LD_{50}, for the amount of HEOD applied, increases dramatically for heavier larvae (Fig. 6-1). Caterpillars that weighed 80 mg needed only

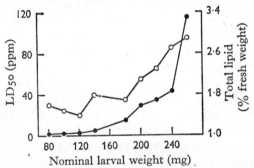

Fig. 6-1. Graph for fifth instar caterpillars of the small tortoiseshell butterfly to show how the toxicity of dieldrin and the percentage of body fat change with caterpillar weight. ○—○, concentration of total fats; ●—●, LD_{50} for dieldrin. (Data from F. Moriarty, 1968.)

0.15 micrograms (μg) of HEOD, whereas caterpillars that weighed 240 mg needed 10.5 μg: a three-fold increase in body weight necessitated a seventy-fold increase in the amount of insecticide applied, or a twenty three-fold increase per unit of body weight.

Not all of the applied insecticide penetrates the cuticle. Whilst it remains on the surface it is physiologically inert. Virtually all the dieldrin that penetrated the cuticle was absorbed within 24 hours of application, and it was found that 24 hours after application the heavier caterpillars contained a lower proportion of their dose of applied insecticide than did the lighter caterpillars. However, dieldrin toxicity was still less for the heavier caterpillars after due allowance had been made for the lower percentage absorption and greater weight of tissue. The amount of HEOD found within the body 24 hours after dosing can be expressed as a fraction of the body weight when dosed. This gives an index for the concentration of absorbed insecticide, and is larger for the heavier caterpillars. On this basis, when 80 mg caterpillars are compared with 240 mg caterpillars, the amount of dieldrin absorbed per unit of body weight only increases fourteen-fold.

The most likely explanation for this considerable decrease in acute toxicity is the increase in fat reserves (Fig. 6-1). Insects have a very discontinuous pattern of growth, with alternate periods of eating and moulting. The last, fifth, instar caterpillar of small tortoiseshell butterflies lays down considerable fat reserves, which are used to carry the insect through the pupal, non-feeding, stage to the adult instar. By analogy, from studies on vertebrates, we may suppose that the highest concentrations of HEOD will be found in these fat reserves. So when the fat reserves increase, less HEOD is available for the site of action. It does appear, from the limited evidence available, that when insects increase their fat reserves their resistance to the fat-soluble organochlorine insecticides also increases. One must be careful however, not to extend this idea to make comparisons between species. It is not true to suggest that the species with more fat reserves will therefore be more resistant to organochlorine insecticides.

This account indicates the various shades of meaning which can be attached to the term 'dose'. In the example above, the simplest meaning is the total quantity of insecticide applied to the insect's surface. Physiologically we are interested in the amount that actually penetrates the body. Even if the dose is taken orally, or is injected into the body, the situation may be complicated. Ingestion does not necessarily guarantee absorption from the gut into the body—at the crudest level the animal may vomit the dose out again. And the availability of compounds such as DDT, which are insoluble in water, after injection is difficult to assess. DDT can be injected dissolved in olive oil, when it is not available to the organism until released from the oil. If injected in a solvent that mixes with blood, the insecticide is likely to precipitate out within the body.

There is another important limit to the relevance of LD_{50}s. An LD_{50} only assesses the risk of death, but other, sublethal, deleterious effects may also occur.

So, to return to our main theme, once we had found the lethal doses of dieldrin and DDT for fifth instar caterpillars of small tortoiseshell butterflies, it was then possible to observe the survivors for sublethal effects. If insecticides had affected the number of small tortoiseshell butterflies by their direct effects on this species, there were, in general terms, three ways in which they could have done it. They could affect the individual's chances of survival: this need not necessarily be by abrupt death from insecticide poisoning. Sublethal effects that reduce the individual's survival abilities could also be significant. Secondly, insecticides could also affect individual's reproductive capacities, or, finally, they could affect the genetic constitution of future generations. On the tentative assumption that any sublethal effect is deleterious, the immediate question resolves itself into this: what is the smallest dose that will produce a sublethal effect? This is a difficult question to answer, but it is important that we try. I shall start by discussing, for *Aglais urticae*, the lowest concentrations for which we have experimental evidence of sublethal effects.

We found that dieldrin given to the fifth, last instar, caterpillars can produce sterile adults:

Amount of dieldrin applied to larvae (μg)	Number of egg clumps laid by five pairs of adults	Total number of eggs laid	Fertile eggs (%)
0	12	1 344	84
1.25	2	146	84
5.0	2	18	0
20.0	0	0	0

We also know the amount of dieldrin present in the body from the time of dosing until after the adults emerge. But we do not know at what stage the dieldrin starts the chain of events which leads to sterility. The rudiments of the reproductive organs are present in the fifth instar caterpillars, so the initial damage could occur at any time from the moment of dosing onwards. So in this instance we have little idea of the effective concentration of dieldrin necessary for sterility to occur. There was however one instance where we could make a guess at the effective concentration.

Adult survivors were abnormally active if they had been dosed, as caterpillars, with 5 μg or more of dieldrin. This behaviour resembled the typical pattern of hyperactivity associated with the early symptoms of poisoning, and it is a reasonable presumption that this aberrant behaviour was caused by the dieldrin present at that time, which was about 1–3 ppm. This figure must be accepted with some caution. The relevant measurement is the concentration of dieldrin at the site of action, whereas we are measuring the whole body concentration. And this is likely to depend largely on the amount of fat reserves in the body, as we have already seen for acute toxicity.

However, we decided to take 1 ppm of dieldrin in the whole body as the critical concentration. Greater amounts would suggest the possibility of deleterious effects, whereas lesser amounts would probably indicate no risk to the organism. This was an arbitrary decision, based on inadequate data, and I have already indicated some of the necessary qualifications. For the moment however let us accept this figure of 1 ppm.

Small tortoiseshells rapidly convert absorbed DDT to DDE. Both DDE and dieldrin are reasonably persistent in this species so, if field specimens of small tortoiseshells were chronically exposed to these two insecticides there was a reasonable expectation that chemical analysis of such specimens would detect these residues. Two tests were made. In the first, twenty-two newly-emerged adults were caught on agricultural land near Holme Fen National Nature Reserve in Huntingdonshire. For the second test, caterpillars were placed on nettles at various distances from the edge of a 1½-acre plot of brussels sprouts, which was then sprayed with DDT, by hand lance, at the rate of ¾ lb/acre. The caterpillars were collected three days later—the nearest group were ten yards from the edge of the plot. In neither test could any organochlorine insecticide residues be detected in the specimens, and the limit of detection was less than 0.01 ppm. This contrasts strongly with the figure of at least 1 ppm needed to produce any effect, and we concluded that, outside of sprayed areas, it was unlikely that insecticides were affecting British butterflies. This conclusion was tentative: in particular we had no information on possible effects on earlier stages in the life cycle, we could not be sure we had noticed all the deleterious effects, and these results were obtained from only one species.

However, it was the best evidence available, and so we suggested that if the number of butterflies has decreased in Britain, it is not because of organochlorine insecticides. It now seems that one important factor is loss of suitable habitat. Where conditions are suitable for a species, then numbers are, by and large, as high as ever. Considerable fluctuations do occur from year to year, and the chief determinant appears to be how sunny the weather is during the period of mating and egg-laying. For example, J. P. Dempster concluded from a brief study of the small copper butterfly (*Lycaena phlaeas*) that it had probably become scarcer in eastern England during the mid-1960s because of reduced sunshine (Fig. 6-2). Females of this species only lay eggs in sunny conditions: 1969 was sunny, and the numbers of this butterfly increased again. The numbers of some species are changing of course, but these changes appear to be part of the normal pattern of ecological change, quite unaffected by pollutants.

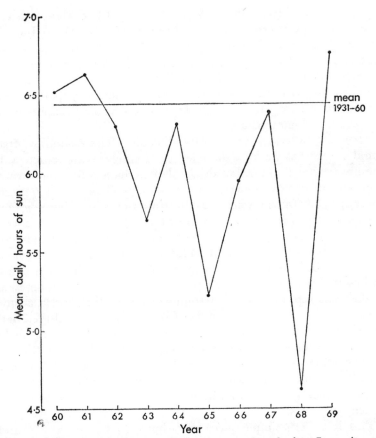

Fig. 6-2. Mean number of hours sunshine per day during June–August, 1960-1969, in eastern England, compared with the mean value for the previous thirty years. (Data from J. P. Dempster, 1971.)

In general, two approaches are possible in the search for sublethal effects. One may either make an empirical approach, or a more fundamental one derived from knowledge of the primary lesion.

The usual, empirical, way is to observe individuals who, either by accident or design, have been exposed to a specific pollutant, and look for any unusual features. We have already discussed several of the symptoms that organochlorine insecticides can produce: thin eggshells, reduced fertility, aberrant behaviour.

One complication is that the interval between dose and response may vary. When symptoms appear must depend, to a large extent, on the amount of insecticide at the site of action. The highest concentrations of insecticide are usually found in the fatty tissues. If starved, an animal uses up its fat reserves, when much insecticide returns to the blood stream and amounts in other parts of the body tend to increase. R. F. Bernard, in the USA, showed about ten years ago that house sparrows that had been dosed with DDT, but were apparently normal, developed symptoms of poisoning when starved. Shortage of food is not all that uncommon, and many animals have stages in their lives when they have naturally to mobilise their fat reserves: insects use fat reserves for energy during pupation, many animals hibernate, and some birds fly considerable distances during migration without feeding.

There is another, more serious, difficulty. The examples of sub-lethal effects that we have discussed are relatively easy to detect, but one always has the nagging doubt that perhaps other, more subtle, effects have been overlooked. The effect of DDT on a simple piece of housefly behaviour may serve to illustrate the point. Houseflies have to extend their proboscis before they can imbibe liquids. A housefly can be stimulated to extend its proboscis if some of its chemosensory hairs are exposed to a suitable solution, such as sucrose. Obviously there must be a minimum concentration of sucrose below which the proboscis is not extended. Two American workers, S. A. Soliman and L. K. Cutkomp, put known amounts of DDT, dissolved in acetone, onto the body surface of house flies (*Musca domestica*) and then determined the minimum sucrose concentration which was needed to elicit extension of the proboscis. They found that the threshold concentration decreased five or six fold with a dose of DDT which was about $1/350$ of the LD_{50} dose, and which was about $\frac{1}{8}$ of the dose needed to kill some flies and about $\frac{1}{4}$ of the dose needed to produce visible symptoms.

This is a very simple piece of behaviour, but even so, careful attention to details, such as age of flies and method of giving stimuli, is essential for reproducible results. The more complicated the behaviour, the more difficult it is likely to be to detect any effects of pollutants, even if they occur.

This puts us into the position where we have to say: we could not detect any effects by such and such a pollutant below a certain degree of exposure, and we looked for effects on the following systems. But of course there is always the possibility of an effect on some other bodily function that we did not examine.

This is rather unsatisfactory, and there is no very obvious way out of the problem. However, the primary lesion may give us some help in deciding which bodily functions to study. For example, DDT affects the nervous system, so one might suppose that this will be the first system to be affected. It may be no coincidence that the effect of DDT on proboscis extension has probably been obtained at as low a dose, relative to the LD_{50} dose, as any other effect by an insecticide observed so far. Surprisingly little use has been made of this approach so far, so we cannot yet decide how useful an idea it is, but it does of course rest on at least two important assumptions. The first is that the pollutant has only one effective primary lesion. It is quite likely that a pollutant may produce several lesions, but if one of these is lethal at concentrations below those needed for the others, the others will only be of academic interest. In principle perhaps it should not make much odds if there is in fact more than one primary lesion, but how do we know how many primary lesions there are? The details of one lesion can, with luck, be worked out from studies with large doses, when the effects should be relatively easy to discover. But it may be much more difficult to distinguish a second lesion from the secondary effects of the first lesion.

The other assumption is that the metabolites have no effect. Sometimes, if the metabolic pathways are known, this can be checked by tests with the metabolites.

We are only now just beginning to investigate these problems, and there is little more that can usefully be said at present. Official reports repeatedly stress the need for more studies on the biological effects of pollutants on wildlife, and this really is the crucial question, which tends to become obscured by the numerous data on residues in both the physical environment and within organisms. Residue data are not an end in themselves, but a means of deciding whether specific pollutants are likely to have adverse effects. Too often we cannot say what is the biological significance of residue data.

So far we have implicitly assumed that all sublethal effects are deleterious. This assumption became particularly acute when it was discovered that organochlorine insecticides could stimulate enzyme induction. This is a perfectly normal phenomenon in vertebrates, where it occurs for the most part only in the liver. Compounds absorbed from the gut pass first to the liver, which is a major site for processing and distribution. It has been shown during the last two decades that many drugs and chemicals found in the environment, including PCBs and organochlorine insecticides, stimulate, or induce, the liver to synthesise more of the enzymes that metabolise them. This can be regarded as an adaptive response by the animal—the induced enzymes metabolise these foreign compounds into forms that are more easily excreted. There is one complication: these enzymes are not specific to the compounds that induce their production. In particular, enzymes induced by PCBs and organochlorine insecticides also metabolise the animal's endogenous steroid hormones, of which the most widely known are probably the male and female sex hormones. Many fears have been expressed that such induction by foreign compounds would disrupt the normal hormone balance. The immediate answer must be that if more than usual amounts of the steroid hormones are being metabolised in the liver then the animal will respond by an increased output of these hormones to maintain the appropriate concentrations in the body. It must also be accepted however that we have, at present, insufficient evidence to decide that such changes are of no physiological significance.

My own attitude can best be illustrated by the results of an experiment by two American workers, J. E. Wergedal and A. E. Harper, published in 1964. It should first be explained that some nutrients, as well as foreign compounds, can also stimulate enzyme induction. Rats were allocated to two groups. One group was fed on a diet with a high protein content, whilst the other group was fed on a diet with a low protein content. Proteins are of course an essential component of most animals' diet, and during digestion they are broken down into their constituent amino-acids, of which the simplest is glycine. After the rats had been fed on these diets for from five to twenty days, they were starved for twelve hours. Each rat was then given a single injection of glycine, when all the rats previously fed on a high protein diet died, whilst half of those on a low protein diet survived. The explanation was quite simple. The high protein diet induced rats to produce more of the enzymes that metabolise amino-acids, when ammonia is formed as a by-product. Ammonia is highly toxic, and is usually metabolised to urea, which is then excreted. When the rats were injected with glycine, those that had been fed on a high protein diet metabolised it more rapidly, and so produced ammonia more rapidly. Normally this would have presented no problems, but because the rats had been starved they lacked the intermediate compounds needed for the conversion of ammonia to the much less toxic urea.

The moral I wish to draw from this tale is quite simple. Enzyme induction is an adaptive response, but it is possible to conceive of circumstances when the response works to the animal's disadvantage. Agreed that an injection of glycine is, in normal circumstances, a most unlikely event for any rat to encounter, but I do not think this invalidates the deduction, that an adaptive response might, in some situations, actually be disadvantageous. I would tentatively conclude that enzyme induction by the organochlorine insecticides is not to be interpreted as a deleterious effect. Of course, a Jeremiah might conclude that, because life depends on the continual avoidance of risks, the safest thing to do is to die—then there are no more problems to cope with.

This question of what constitutes a deleterious response is particularly acute for our own species, when we are concerned for the welfare of each and every individual. Not only are there the difficulties, already discussed, of deciding when deleterious effects occur.

In addition, as we saw with the LD_{50}, different individuals give different degrees of response to the same exposure. This implies that, given a large enough number of individuals, a very small proportion of them may be adversely affected by exposures much smaller than those necessary for the rest of the population. The empirical approach is to decide, from the available evidence, the critical degree of exposure or critical level of residue concentration above which damage is likely to occur. A safety factor is then used, commonly of one hundred-fold, to set an acceptable daily intake (A.D.I.) or similar standard.

This vexatious problem has caused much debate with radioactive nuclides. Massive acute doses, such as occurred at Hiroshima, cause rapid deaths, but the usual potential hazards are rather more insidious. Damage occurs because radiation from such nuclides can disrupt cells: both body cells and germ cells. Effects commonly become manifest either as cancers, which may take years to develop, or as genetic effects in future generations. Such events have to be regarded in terms of probabilities: the probability increases as the exposure increases, and is affected greatly by the individual's age at the time of the exposure. It becomes very difficult to decide what exposure will produce somatic effects in, say, one individual out of ten thousand. Such predictions can only be made by extrapolation from the knowledge we have about the risks from larger doses. Extrapolations are notoriously unreliable, and the standard custom has long been to suppose that probability of effect is directly related to exposure, and to assume that any degree of exposure will increase the probability of damage. One could argue from the available evidence that there is a threshold degree of radiation below which no damage occurs, but practical policies are based on the more cautious assumption.

Decisions have to be taken when, for example, a new nuclear power station is designed. How much radioactive effluent can we permit to be released into the environment? One approach is 'cost benefit analysis', in which all costs and all benefits have to be expressed in money terms. The aim, which is laudable, is to decide rationally how much release will confer the maximum benefit, which is that degree of control at which the cost of reducing effluent release any further becomes more expensive than the value of the additional benefits achieved by the additional reduction. The legitimacy of this exercise must depend on how effectively one can, for example, quote a price for increasing the probability of leukaemia by 0.001 %. Obviously there is a need for careful thought and debate, but it might be more convincing if this type of analysis were confined, as it sometimes is, to those items that can reasonably be given monetary values, with a separate inventory of all the less easily evaluated consequences. This way the public should be given the relevant information on which a decision has to be based: arbitrary monetary values for, say, an increased incidence of leukaemia, may not be generally acceptable.

The emphasis so far in this chapter has been on the effects of pollutants on individual organisms, although the initial question was about the effects of insecticides on populations. For conservation, and many other practical purposes, we are only concerned with the size of populations, not with the fate of individual animals. The transition from individual to population of individuals introduces additional complexities of interpretation.

This is not the place for a detailed analysis of the factors that determine population size, but two simple facts are worth noting. Most animal populations have a very high potential reproductive rate, so that the population will grow rapidly unless a large proportion of the offspring dies before they reproduce. In fact, most populations maintain fairly constant numbers in the long run, although there may be considerable fluctuations within relatively short periods of time. Pollutants are an additional potential cause of death, but few detailed studies have been made of the ways in which they may affect populations. In fact most of our information derives from studies on the effects of insecticides on pest species, but the principles should apply to many other species and pollutants too. One may be forgiven for supposing that a pollutant can only reduce the size of populations. I shall give examples of three other types of response by populations: resurgence, increase in numbers, and genetic change.

Work by J. P. Dempster, at Monks Wood, gave a very clear illustration of resurgence: DDT at first reduced the size of a population, but it then became larger than it would have been if no DDT had ever been used. One of the principal pests of brussels sprouts is the small cabbage white butterfly (*Pieris rapae*), whose caterpillars feed on the plants until they wander off to pupate. Normally there are two generations each year. Each summer from 1964–1966 an experimental plot of brussels sprouts was sprayed twice with DDT, at about the times when there were maximum numbers of first or second generation caterpillars on the plants. The DDT gave a very good kill of the caterpillars that were on the plants at the time of spraying, but, although DDT is persistent, the effects did not last very long. After the first application of DDT each summer, the number of second generation eggs laid on the brussels sprouts was comparable with the number laid on plants in a similar control, unsprayed, plot. These plots were small, only a quarter of an acre, so that ovipositing females were easily able to come in from other areas. Differences of plant growth were the main reason for any differences of egg numbers between the sprayed and unsprayed plots. Moreover, the second generation eggs were laid on newly expanded young leaves, and the caterpillars fed on these young leaves until, later, they moved into the hearts of the plants. This meant, as the plants were growing rapidly, that the second generation on the sprayed plots was little affected by the residues from the first spray of DDT, and was able to develop satisfactorily. However, the survival figures for second generation eggs and caterpillars, from the start of this generation until the plants were sprayed a second time, are rather surprising:

	Number of eggs laid on sampled plants		Total mortality of eggs and caterpillars (%)	
Year	Unsprayed	Sprayed	Unsprayed	Sprayed
1964	424	418	73.9	63.3
1965	184	223	57.1	29.8
1966	724	442	67.3	53.6

Eggs laid on plants in the sprayed plot had a better chance of surviving—until the second spray—than had the eggs on the unsprayed plot. This increased survival occurred because there were fewer predators, which killed fewer caterpillars. The principal predators were arthropods such as harvestmen (*Phalangidae*) and ground-beetles (*Carabidae*) that dwell most of their time on the ground, where they were continually exposed to residues of DDT. Thus differences of behaviour between predators and their prey meant that the DDT affected the predators more than the prey species.

This example shows very clearly that the net results of a non-specific poison on a population can be complex. Even in the simpler situation, where a pollutant only affects one species, it is difficult to predict the effects on population size. If some individuals are killed by the pollutant, fewer may die from other causes.

Red spider mite is the classic example of the next type of response: a species increasing in numbers because of insecticides. It had been known for some decades that these mites occur, in very low numbers, in orchards. They became a serious pest soon after DDT was first used in orchards. This mite is not easily affected by DDT, and the standard explanation for the increase is that DDT kills the predators that normally control the number of mites. It must be admitted that the evidence to support this explanation is incomplete. It has been shown experimentally that DDT can improve the nutrient value of plants on which the mite feeds, so that the mites produce more offspring. This may be a contributory factor. For our purposes however the details are not too important. The important and undisputed fact is that DDT can increase the population of red spider mites.

Finally we come to genetic changes within a population. Already by the late 1940s reports were coming in from various parts of the world that first houseflies, and then other insect pests, were becoming resistant to DDT. Since then populations of an ever increasing number of species have developed resistance to many insecticides. This resistance does not develop by changes within individual insects, but by selection (survival) of those individuals within a population that are already more resistant to the insecticide than are the rest. Such a change in a population's genetic constitution only occurs after several, usually many, generations have suffered a high mortality from an insecticide. As might be expected, such populations are not in general as well adapted for survival, except for this better ability to withstand insecticides. The population usually reverts to the original susceptible strain once this selection pressure is removed.

Resistant strains of insects pose many practical problems of great importance. The difficulties are compounded by the fact that not only can one species develop resistance to more than one insecticide, but sometimes resistance to one insecticide automatically increases resistance to some other insecticides. Resistance has also been found in fish, but in general vertebrates are less likely to acquire resistance because the interval between generations is so much longer. However, wherever populations are exposed to a pollutant at a sufficiently high level for long enough, one may expect some genetic shift. Two more rather diverse examples should suffice.

The first harks back to the 'dark satanic mills' of the industrial revolution. Our industrial cities were, at one time, very dark places— everything was covered with soot. So much so that at least one little girl seriously believed that her local town hall was built of coal. Happily this state of affairs is rapidly disappearing, but it did leave its mark on some species of moth. Moths from these industrial areas were markedly darker in colour than those found in less sooty areas. This melanism developed by selection pressure in the same way as resistance to insecticides. Melanic forms were less easily seen by predators in these industrial areas than were moths with the normal colouring. In recent years the degree of pollution has decreased in many of our industrial towns and cities, and R. R. Askew *et al* have shown that in Manchester this has been accompanied by a decrease in the proportion of melanic forms.

Our final example also comes from an activity that flourished with the development of the industrial revolution—mining for metals. Old mine sites frequently have piles of waste material left after most of the metal had been extracted. Few species of plant can grow in such places. Not only are there the residues of toxic metals, but also essential nutrients are often in short supply. However, a few species do survive here, and again it has been found that these populations are tolerant of the conditions, have developed by selection from normal populations, and are genetically distinct from them.

It is a nice question whether such genetic changes are strictly deleterious. They may be sometimes, because such populations will have a less diverse genetic structure, and therefore be less able to respond to any other environmental changes that may occur.

To conclude, I must mention 'the balance of Nature'. It is sometimes said that this is upset by pollutants. It is difficult to discover precisely what is meant by this term, but it seems to imply that there is only one balance in the numbers of individuals and species, and that it continues forever. In fact each species is continually struggling to survive, and considerable fluctuations do occur from time to time and from place to place in the fortunes of each species, even without the intervention of our own species. Pollutants are merely one more factor amongst a host of others that affect the numbers of plants and animals.

7

Heavy Metals and Radioisotopes

So far we have discussed a limited range of synthetic molecules. I want now to consider the heavy metals, a group of elements which has also achieved some notoriety as pollutants. They are of interest in their own right, but will also serve to illustrate and extend some of the ideas that we have already developed.

The word metal usually suggests an element that exists in the solid state at normal temperatures, and which is dense, ductile, a good conductor of electricity and so on, in contrast to non-metallic elements. There are exceptions to these criteria—the metal mercury for instance is liquid at normal temperatures—but broad similarities do exist between all metals. Heavy metals are commonly taken to include all metals except for those in the first three periods of the periodic table for elements, and it also excludes the alkali and alkaline earth metals. This may not be very meaningful to those with little knowledge of chemistry, but that does not matter unduly. There is no complete consensus of opinion on precisely which elements are heavy metals, different technical dictionaries give different criteria, and in practice the phrase is used as a loose generic term.

Unlike the synthetic organic molecules, metals occur naturally in the physical environment. It is no great surprise then that organisms have a definite need for many metals. For example, zinc occurs in the enzyme carbonic anhydrase, which we discussed in chapter four, cobalt is in vitamin B_{12}, iron in haemoglobin, copper in other respiratory pigments. Vanadium is an interesting oddity, not found in most animals but concentrated by ascidians (sea squirts) more than half a million times above the level in the ambient sea water. Its function is unknown. So we have the situation where a lack of these metals can cause deficiency diseases, whilst too much can be toxic.

We will restrict our attention to two heavy metals, lead and mercury, which have no known biological functions, although traces can be found in most organisms, and which are well known as pollutants.

Lead was probably the first serious pollutant: it has been suggested as the prime cause for the decline and fall of the Roman Empire. Clearly it must be very difficult to prove this assertion, but the known facts make a plausible argument. It has been estimated that about eight pounds of lead per head of population were used annually in Italy during the first and second centuries AD. This is surprisingly high when compared with recent figures for industrial uses of lead in the USA, which are about twenty pounds per head per annum. Biologically of course, the degree of exposure is far more important than the total amount in use. The Romans used much of their lead for water pipes and in containers for food and drink. Tap water commonly does not dissolve lead from water pipes because of carbonates in the water which form a protective film on the interior of the pipes. However, pure water with carbon dioxide will dissolve lead, and so will organic acids, such as acetic acid (vinegar) or the acids in fruits. So it is reasonable to suppose that those Romans wealthy enough to afford leaden storage utensils had a high exposure to lead. Certainly we would not tolerate the sale of leaden utensils now, because of the risk of poisoning. Lead has been found in human bones of that period, but not from earlier and later periods, which does help to corroborate the suggestion.

Lead has therefore a long history of use by man. Its attractions include a low melting point $(327°C)$, which means that it is extracted easily from its ores. It is also easily worked, and resistant to water and many acids. It is unfortunately also very persistent within organisms, and toxic. Present evidence suggests that the amounts of lead in the environment have increased considerably, as a result of man's activities.

Residues of pollutants, such as lead, that also occur naturally offer an additional difficulty of interpretation which does not occur with synthetic pollutants—it can be difficult to decide what proportion of any particular residue is due to man's activities. It has been estimated that air contains, from natural processes, about 0.0005 μg of lead/metre^3 of air, which has been derived, as airborne dust and by gaseous diffusion, from the earth's crust. M. Murozumi *et al* got some interesting relevant data by analysing ice samples from Greenland and Antarctica. These ice sheets never melt, and so the annual layers of precipitation can be distinguished and dated. Thus it is possible, with painstaking techniques to avoid contamination, to measure the concentration of elements in the precipitation from previous centuries. Greenland ice deposited in 800 BC contains less than 0.001 pp10^9 of lead. This had increased by 1750 AD, which is about the start of the Industrial Revolution, to 0.011 pp10^9. There has been a fairly steady rate of increase ever since (Fig. 7-1). Murozumi *et al* concluded from their data that there was a steady rise in the amount of lead until about 1940, after which there was an abrupt increase in the rate at which concentrations rose. They attributed this to a change at about that time in the significant sources of lead in the air. Personally I doubt whether the data show much evidence of a

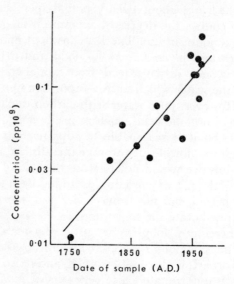

Fig. 7-1. Increasing concentrations of lead in samples from the Greenland ice sheet. Note the geometric scale on the vertical axis. (Data from M. Morozumi, T. J. Chow & C. Patterson, 1969.)

sudden change in the rate of increase at that time, but certainly the sources of lead changed. Until 1940, most of this lead had escaped into the air from the smelting of lead ores, when very fine particles pass into suspension in the air to form an aerosol, which could then be dispersed far and wide. From 1750 to 1880, perhaps 2% of refined lead was lost in this way. Subsequent improvements of technique have now reduced this figure to about 0.06%. It is then possible to estimate the amount of lead released as an aerosol from smelting into the northern hemisphere, and to compare this with the amount of lead found in the Greenland ice:

Year	Lead aerosols produced from smelting (tons × 10^3)	Lead in Greenland ice (pp 10^9)
1753	2	0.01
1815	4	0.03
1933	8	0.07
1966	2	0.2

The two sets of values clearly correlate very well except for the most recent date. However, the major source of lead in the atmosphere today is from car exhaust fumes:

Year	Lead aerosols produced from exhaust fumes (tons $\times 10^3$)	Total lead aerosols produced (tons $\times 10^3$)
1753	—	2
1815	—	4
1933	4	12
1966	100	102

We will consider aerial transport of pollutants in chapter nine, but it should be appreciated that correlations between concentrations of lead in Greenland ice and amounts emitted are likely to vary with time—both climate and smelting sites change. The importance of site is emphasised by the fact that lead in ice from Antarctica was below the limits of detection until 1940, after which it reached about 0.02 $pp10^9$, a tenth of the concentration found in the Greenland ice samples.

The Greenland and Antarctic ice data are probably the best available for assessing how man's activities have increased the concentrations of lead, but there are also some other clues. Deep oceanic waters (more than 1,000 metres below the surface) appear to be unaffected, with about 0.02–0.04 $pp10^9$ of lead, but surface waters in the Mediterranean and Pacific now contain ten times as much. There is at least one example of a similar increase in biological material. Amounts of lead in mosses from Skane, in Sweden, have quadrupled during the last century. One other revealing statistic—air over the largest American cities contains 2,000 times, and air in sparsely populated rural areas 100 times, as much lead as air over the mid-Pacific. Most of this airborne lead must come from man's activities, and the presumption is that most of it derives from car exhausts. Tetra-ethyl lead is added to petrol to prevent premature combustion, and it is undoubtedly an important source of lead in town air, although it is rapidly broken down by light and heat to other forms. An inventory made in 1968 in the USA showed that over 98% of all lead emitted into the air came from the combustion of petrol, although this 'does not include attrition of the innumerable lead-containing items that are subject to weathering and often are burned or otherwise disposed of after they have outlived their usefulness', and which may be an important additional source.

We can summarise what we know about the movement of lead in the environment by a simple flow chart:

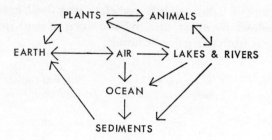

We lack vital information on the chemical forms, amounts and rates of transfer for lead in most parts of the environment, but we do know that the lead in the atmosphere is replaced on average every one to four weeks. Much of the lead in vehicle exhaust fumes that is attached to particles settles out from the air within a few hundred feet of the roadway, where it may form an appreciable deposit on plant surfaces.

The really important question of course is, what effects does lead have on living organisms? Answers can verge on the bizarre. It was estimated in 1969 that a million ducks, geese and swans die each year in the USA from lead poisoning. About 6,000 tons of lead shot are fired at water fowl each year, much of it ends up at the bottom of the lakes and rivers, and some of this spent lead shot is then eaten by waterfowl when searching for gravel. Less surprisingly, fish have been eliminated from rivers that have been contaminated by lead, and other metals, from old mine workings.

One might be inclined to suggest though that man is the principal species endangered by lead, because the highest emissions of lead occur in densely populated areas. However, lead in the air appears to be a relatively minor source of the residues in our bodies, although there is some uncertainty about this because we do not yet know enough about the fate of inhaled lead. Food and water appear to be the main sources of lead for man, with, in Great Britain, an average daily intake of about 200 μg from food, and perhaps an additional 20 μg from water. Net absorption from the gut is about 5–10% of the intake, so an average adult will acquire about 10–20 μg of lead per day from food and drink.

About 95% of the lead in man occurs in the bones, which are to lead what adipose tissue is to DDT, a storage site. Whilst lead remains in bone tissue it is, so far as we know, physiologically inert—unless it is a radioactive isotope—and it is only slowly released. Lead is also taken up into bone rather slowly, and there are some data to suggest that the amount of lead in bone tissue increases up to and perhaps beyond the age of forty, although there is no concurrent increase in blood concentrations.

Lead poisoning does not result from an effect at one specific site. Biochemical lesions occur in a range of enzymes that can combine strongly with lead and are then less active. There is some evidence to suggest that enzymes associated with membranes are particularly vulnerable. This type of lesion is rather different from that of DDT, which affects one specific activity, the conduction of nerve impulses. DDT may cause other lesions, but they would appear to be few in number, whereas lead can affect directly many different enzymes. So it is no surprise to find that several organs are affected, and effects on the kidneys, nervous system and formation of haemoglobin are relatively well understood. We shall confine ourselves to the effects on haemoglobin synthesis.

Haemoglobin of course is the pigment that gives blood its red colour. It occurs within the red blood corpuscles, is essential for the transport of oxygen from the lungs to all parts of the body, and is also essential for the transport of carbon dioxide from the tissues and for the regulation of blood pH (degree of acidity or alkalinity). It consists of a protein, globin, united with the pigment haem. Haem is synthesised by a series of chemical reactions, and lead affects enzymes involved in at least three stages of this process. The clinical result is anaemia, and it is also possible to detect increased amounts of some of the intermediate compounds. The intermediate of greatest interest is ALA (δ-aminolevulinic acid), which is normally transformed to porphobilinogen (PBG) by the enzyme ALAD (ALA dehydrase). Lead inhibits ALAD, ALA therefore accumulates, and it can be detected in blood serum and in urine.

It would be convenient if the concentration of lead in the blood were a reliable indicator for the severity of any toxic effects: blood samples can be taken easily and with minimal risk of adverse effects. Unfortunately this is not always so. Similar blood levels can be associated with very different degrees of poisoning. There is the additional minor complication that most of the lead in the blood is associated with red blood cells, lead causes anaemia, so the number of cells decreases. It is not obvious what is the most satisfactory measure for the amount of lead in the blood.

In practice, for children, lead concentrations in the blood of more than 0.6 ppm (commonly expressed as 60 μg/100 g whole blood) are taken to indicate lead poisoning if other data, such as anaemia, corroborate it. For adults, 0.8 ppm is taken as the critical level, above which clear-cut symptoms of lead poisoning can be expected. This figure is based almost entirely on men who are otherwise healthy, but who have obtained high blood levels from their work. We need more information about mild degrees of poisoning, and about interactions with other stresses: the normal range of values for lead in blood is 0.1–0.4 ppm, which is rather close to the critical level.

Obviously we need a measure for the amount of lead in the body that correlates well with its adverse effects. A standard method in current use is to remove lead from the body by administering a chelating agent (calcium ethylene diamine tetra acetate), which sequesters some of the readily available lead. It is then excreted in the urine and the amount can be measured. The amount so excreted is not directly proportional to the total amount of lead in the body— the amount excreted after any degree of exposure decreases as the time since exposure increases. The presumption is that, with time, more and more of the lead in the body is stored in the bone. The hope is that the amount of lead excreted after treatment with a chelating agent reflects the amounts readily mobilised in the body and, in particular, of the amounts at the sites of action. P. B. Hammond attempted to test this. He took, as his index of toxicity, the degree of inhibition of ALAD in the liver. We do not fully understand the toxicological significance of ALAD inhibition, but inhibition does increase the amount of ALA in the blood, and excessive amounts are excreted in the urine. He found, for experimental rats, that when the amount of lead excreted is plotted on a geometric scale the activity is linearly related to the ALAD activity of the liver (Fig. 7-2). It must

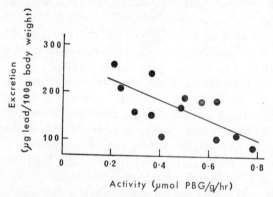

Fig. 7-2. Rate of activity of ALAD in the rat liver and the amount of lead excreted after treatment with a chelating agent. (Reproduced, modified, from P. B. Hammond, 1973.)

be admitted that there was a considerable degree of scatter for individual values about the best fitting line, but this could reflect the normal variation in ALAD activity between rats. This relationship held after both a single large dose of lead was infused, and after it had been imbibed with drinking water for five to eight days. One can conclude then that, if ALAD activity in the liver is a fair measure of toxicity, then the degree of lead poisoning can be assessed by seeing how much lead is excreted after treatment with a chelating agent. This presumption is probably reasonable: ALA excretion in urine correlates well with the symptoms of lead poisoning.

The emphasis so far in this chapter has been on our own species, although the general ideas should apply to a wide range of organisms. I would like to mention just two aspects about lead in wildlife.

A large amount of the lead in birds occurs in their bone too, but feathers are probably an equally important site. J. L. F. Parslow *et al* found that about 35 % of the lead in puffins (*Fratercula arctica*) was in the feathers, which are replaced annually. This is therefore, in effect, a way of excreting lead.

One could reasonably suppose, since lead is so persistent within organisms, that it would concentrate up the food chain. By and large this may well be the case, but not always. R. B. Holtzman studied a very simple food chain in the Arctic. Sedge and lichen grow very slowly in the adverse environment, and so acquire high concentrations of lead deposited from the air. Reindeer feed substantially on this vegetation. Their predator the wolf has lower concentrations of lead than they do. The explanation is simple. Most of the lead in the reindeer is in the bones, but wolves only eat the flesh, not the bones. So the wolf's feeding behaviour minimises its exposure to lead in its prey.

Mercury became prominent as a serious pollutant when the cause of Minamata disease was discovered. Minamata Bay, in Japan, has several small villages along its shore, with a total population of about 10,000. From 1953 to 1960 nearly 100 people, mostly inhabitants of these villages, developed what came to be called Minamata disease. The symptoms indicated impairment of the nervous system, and included, in different patients, deafness, blurred vision, unco-ordinated movements, and loss of emotional control. Many died.

The first fifty-two patients, from forty families, were compared with sixty-eight control, unaffected, neighbouring families. This comparison suggested that the disease was associated with the eating of fish and shellfish from Minamata Bay: twenty-five out of the forty affected families ate fish or shellfish from Minamata Bay every day, whereas only five of the control families ate it every day. Moreover, many cats and fish-eating birds were similarly affected. Strong evidence for this suggestion came from animals that were deliberately fed fish from Minamata Bay and then developed the symptoms of this disease.

Many possibilities were considered, but eventually it was concluded that the food was contaminated with mercury. There were high concentrations of mercury both in the mud and in shellfish from Minamata Bay, and in the tissues of patients who had died. The mercury came from a chemical plant that used mercuric chloride as a catalyst in the production of vinyl chloride from acetylene. The crude vinyl chloride was washed to get rid of impurities, which included mercury, and about 60 g of mercury were lost per ton of vinyl chloride produced. Over 300 Kg of mercury were lost this way annually, but it was not clear in what form the mercury was ingested. The amounts of mercury found in patients were insufficient, as mercuric chloride, to have produced overt symptoms, but the symptoms were consistent with poisoning by mercury in an organic form. It was not clear whether this conversion from an inorganic to an organic compound of mercury occurred within the manufacturing plant or after its release into Minamata Bay.

One has to be careful, when discussing the toxicity of elemental pollutants, to consider the different molecular forms in which they can occur. With luck, pollutants such as DDT, whose toxicity depends on the structure of the whole molecule, lose their toxicity when metabolised. At the least, analytically, one can measure how much DDT is present. This is not the situation with pollutants such as mercury. The total amount of mercury in a biological specimen can be determined reliably, with good sensitivity, by atomic absorption or neutron activation. But mercury can occur in many different forms, which differ both in physical and chemical properties, and in their toxicity. Apart from elemental mercury, mercury can form two distinct groups of inorganic compounds. The atom of mercury combines, in mercurous compounds, with a single atom or group, whereas in mercuric compounds it combines with two atoms or groups. All organic mercury compounds have two groups attached to the atom.

Methyl mercury is the form of greatest danger to our own species, and it was subsequently found to be the cause of Minamata disease. In part its toxicity is due to the ease with which it can cross the placenta and accumulate in unborn children, its considerable persistence within organisms, and its affinity for the central nervous system.

Extensive further information has come from Sweden, which has a considerable problem of pollution by mercury. The Swedes have not, so far as is known, had anybody suffer from Minamata disease, although some individuals without symptoms have had higher residue levels than some of the Japanese victims. A rook (*Corvus frugilegus*) provided the first recorded case of poisoning, in 1950, and later that decade several bird populations declined drastically in numbers. During later studies feathers were analysed from museum specimens of several bird species, and specimens before 1940 contained far less mercury than later ones. For example, G. Birke *et al* analysed tail feathers from the goshawk (*Accipiter gentilis*):

Period	Mean concentration of mercury (*ppm*)
1863–1946	2.2
1947–1965	29

From these and other investigations it was eventually concluded that the main source of mercury in terrestrial species was seed dressed with methyl mercury dicyanodiamide ('Panogen'), which had been introduced in 1938 for the control of fungal diseases, especially in cereals and sugar beet. Such results caused concern, especially when it was found that terrestrial predators contained higher residues than their prey, and that agricultural products in Sweden contained more mercury than in other European countries. For example, H. Ackefors quotes some comparative data by G. Westöö *et al* for the concentration of mercury (ppm) in Sweden and Denmark:

	Sweden	Denmark
Eggs	0.029	0.004
Pork chops	0.030	0.003
Pig's liver	0.060	0.009
Beef	0.012	0.003

Methyl mercury seed dressings were banned from use early in 1966. The residues in terrestrial wildlife and in agricultural products have decreased since then.

However, the most serious contamination occurred in the water, in the lakes and rivers and, to a lesser extent, the Baltic. Seed dressings were not involved. Here again feathers from aquatic or fish-eating birds show a recent increase in the amounts of mercury, and Swedish workers consider that these data indicate a slow rise in mercury pollution since the start of the industrial revolution in Sweden, about 1890. For example, A. G. Johnels *et al* analysed feathers of the great crested grebe (*Podiceps cristatus*):

Period	Mean concentration of mercury (*ppm*)
1865–1890	5.6
1890–1915	7.0
1915–1940	10.3
1940–1966	13.6

Certainly there has been an increase since 1940. Fish from some lakes and coastal areas now have such high mercury levels (Table 7-1) that it is forbidden to sell them. In general aquatic organisms

Table 7-1. Amounts of mercury in muscle from fish analysed in Sweden during 1965–1967. (From data presented by H. Ackefors, from original paper by G. Birke *et al*, 1967.)

Source	Range of mercury concentrations (*ppm*)	Fish
Off the Swedish coast in the Baltic and Atlantic	0.02–0.11	Various saltwater fish
West coast of Sweden	0.03–0.20 ⎫	Pike, perch, pike-perch,
Baltic coast of Sweden	0.02–2.5 ⎬	vendace
Swedish lakes	0.05–10.0 ⎭	Pike

do naturally contain more mercury than do terrestrial species. For example sea fish caught during the 1930s and 1940s, presumably before much pollution had occurred, contained 0.03–0.16 ppm mercury. By contrast, FAO and WHO, two of the United Nations organisations, recommended for terrestrial food a residue limit of only 0.05 ppm. But the recent levels found in fish in Sweden do indicate a considerable degree of pollution.

This mercury could not have come from agricultural uses. The two most important sources were probably timber mills and chlor-alkali plants. Sweden exports a considerable amount of wood pulp, and from about 1946 phenyl mercury acetate was used as a fungicide to preserve the pulp. It was banned in 1965. Chlor-alkali plants produce chlorine and caustic soda by the electrolysis of sodium chloride solutions—mercury is used as the cathode, and some is lost in factory effluent.

Nearly all the mercury in fish in Sweden is in the toxic methyl mercury form. At first sight this is surprising, because the three main forms released into the waterways have been elemental mercury, inorganic mercuric compounds and phenyl mercury. Phenyl mercury, and some other organic forms, break down readily to inorganic mercuric compounds, and elemental mercury is oxidised to mercuric compounds. These compounds reside principally in the bottom muds, where they can be converted to methyl mercury. The details of this conversion are not yet completely clear, but many micro-organisms can methylate inorganic mercuric compounds, and the rate at which this conversion occurs is probably an index of the degree of microbial activity. Each waterway probably has its own peculiar pattern of activity. For example, in anaerobic conditions hydrogen sulphide is likely to occur in the muds. This will convert mercuric compounds into the relatively insoluble mercuric sulphide, which cannot be methylated. The introduction of oxygen can result in a slow microbial methylation. Sometimes dimethyl mercury may be formed first, which is volatile and fat-soluble. It breaks down to methyl mercury in acid solutions.

One of the more serious aspects of the problem in Sweden is that it will not easily go away. One chlor-alkali plant closed down in 1925, but there are still high concentrations of mercury in the upper sediments of the adjacent lake. Lakes do differ. This one is oligotrophic (has low levels of nutrient salts), has a low sedimentation rate, and therefore the mercury-rich sediments are covered very slowly. Other lakes where mercury release stopped 25 to 30 years ago have mercury buried many inches deep in the sediments, and consequently fish have relatively low concentrations of mercury.

At least four possible cures have been suggested: to cover the mercury-rich sediment with inert material, such as clay; to cover the sediment with a material, such as freshly ground silica, that will absorb mercury; to add sulphide to the water and so form insoluble mercuric sulphide; to raise the pH, so releasing more dimethyl mercury, although this would then contaminate a larger area.

This problem of large persistent residues of mercury in waterways that then contaminate fish is common in industrial countries. Happily it does not appear to be a problem in Great Britain, although this may be because some of our rivers are so polluted by other substances that no fish can survive anyway. It is a problem in North America—in 1970, waterways in thirty-three states of the USA had high levels of methyl mercury, and many areas were closed indefinitely to fishing. Mercury does show that we can no longer, once we have got rid of our waste materials, automatically forget about them. This may be true too for some members of the next group of pollutants.

So far we have considered pollutants of two types. With some, such as p,p'-DDT, toxicity depends on the structure of the whole molecule. With elements such as mercury it is the atom itself that is toxic, although its toxicity can be considerably modified by the particular type of molecule in which the atom occurs. For completeness, we must briefly consider a third type—radioisotopes—that are toxic because the atom is unstable.

To understand radioisotopes we must know a little about the structure of atoms. As a first approximation we may suppose that an atom consists of a nucleus with a precise number of attendant electrons, each of which has a negative charge. The nucleus consists of protons, with a positive charge, and neutrons, which have no charge. The number of protons determines the number of electrons, and these determine the atom's chemical properties, but individual atoms of the same element may have different numbers of neutrons. Such atoms with the same number of protons but different numbers of neutrons are termed isotopes. For example, hydrogen is the simplest of all atoms, with only one proton, and no neutrons. There are however two other isotopes of hydrogen: deuterium contains one neutron, and tritium two. Deuterium, like hydrogen, is a perfectly stable atom, but tritium is not. Unstable atoms, or radioisotopes, transmute themselves spontaneously into new atoms with a different number of protons. These chemical transformations involve the release of both energy and or sub-atomic particles, which can be harmful to living organisms.

Radioisotopes occur naturally in the environment, and by comparison man's contribution so far has been minute—A. Preston *et al* estimate that we have increased the total radioactivity of the oceans by about 0.1 %. This is however an average figure. The major source of artificial radioactivity during the last three decades has been the testing of nuclear weapons in the atmosphere, when fall-out is spread widely over the globe's surface. In future the major source, barring accidents, is likely to be waste products from nuclear reactors: these will be, at least initially, very restricted in their distribution, and so pose the risk of severe local contamination.

Most of the long-lived waste radioisotopes from reactors are stored, in containers on land, but inevitably a small proportion is released to the environment, principally with the water used for cooling and storing the spent rods of fissionable material from nuclear reactors. Different radioisotopes differ in the degree of their toxicity, and plutonium is currently a cause for concern. It is possibly the most toxic of all the elements, quite apart from its radioactivity. Moreover it has a very long half-life, of 24,300 years. We have already discussed, in the previous chapter, the difficulties of deciding on an acceptable degree of exposure to radioisotopes. Waste products in the cooling water from nuclear reactors are discharged, after treatment, onto the sea bed, or else into lakes, rivers or estuaries. Most of these products eventually reach the oceans.

Deleterious effects are avoided by the 'critical path approach'. For this, one has to know how radioisotopes are distributed in the environment after their release. This, combined with knowledge of what people eat, and where they work and spend their leisure time, enables one to estimate the degree of public exposure for any given release of radioisotopes. So limits can be set on the rates and amounts of release of radioisotopes. Essentially this approach rests on the fact that, for all pollutants, the degree of biological effect depends on the degree of exposure, but we have probably gone further, for this group of potential pollutants, in calculating, in precise quantitative terms, the acceptable degree of environmental contamination, than for any other pollutants.

8

The Guillemot Wreck

We have attempted, so far, to develop some general ideas about the effects that single pollutants may have on both individual animals and on populations of animals. To a large extent these ideas have been developed from very artificial laboratory experiments and from rather controlled field situations. Such studies do help us to understand the effects of pollution, but field situations can be more complex—in particular there are likely to be several significant interacting factors. An incident in the Irish Sea in 1969 underlined the importance of interactions and the difficulties of interpreting field situations.

During September 1969 reports came in from the coasts around the Irish Sea of large numbers of dead and dying birds. By the end of November nearly 17,000 corpses were estimated to have been washed up on the coastline, with presumably many more, possibly within the range 50,000–100,000, that sank and decomposed at sea. Nearly all these birds were guillemots (*Uria aalge*). Because of our current concern about environmental matters a great effort was made, by many individuals and organisations, to discover why these birds had died.

The first obvious question was whether this was an abnormal number of deaths. Guillemots spend most of their time at sea, and during December and January they start to congregate near their breeding sites, inaccessible cliff faces. Each female lays one egg, usually in May, which is incubated for about five weeks, and the hatched chick leaves the breeding ledge in July, when two to three weeks old. The chicks cannot fly when they leave, and flutter straight down to the sea from the breeding sites on the cliff face. These birds are then very vulnerable, and dead juveniles are quite commonly found along the coasts during the early autumn. However, the deaths in 1969 were atypical. The numbers were excessively large. Also, over 90% of the dead guillemots examined in one sample were adults. Normally the death rate is highest amongst juveniles during their first year of life.

There are a few records of previous guillemot 'wrecks', or deaths of

H

many birds, from 1856 onwards, which were often associated with stormy weather. Most of the bodies found in the 1969 wreck were washed up after storms in late September, but although these storms were probably the immediate cause of many of the deaths, some dead and dying birds had appeared during the calm weather earlier in the month, which suggests that the storms were only a secondary cause of death. There were other odd features too about this particular incident. Before it was realised that a large number of guillemots were about to die, there were many reports of odd behaviour. Birds were unusually close to the shore, feeble and listless.

Post-mortem examinations revealed some clues, but it is easier to say what the guillemots did not die from than to say for certain what did kill them. Few of the birds had been affected by oil. Nor was there any reason to suppose that either parasites or diseases were responsible for this wreck, although tests for diseases should ideally be made with material from live specimens, or, at least, from specimens that have died recently. Most of the specimens examined had been dead many days. The birds did lack reserve fat, and were on average about 40 % underweight, although it is debatable whether they were just in poor condition or died from starvation. Perhaps the most interesting result was that kidneys and livers had abnormal symptoms that were suggestive of poisoning.

Many analyses were made for many possible pollutants, and the results for three groups deserve mention: a range of elements (mostly metals), organochlorine insecticides and PCBs. The results of such analyses are of course only meaningful when compared with the results to be expected from normal healthy guillemots. This comparison was made by analysing healthy birds, from Northern Ireland and south-west Scotland, shot in late October and in November.

Some, but not all, of the dead birds had unusually high concentrations of several elements in their livers (Table 8-1). In fact the data are reminiscent of those in Table 5-2, where the upper limit for the range of values in birds found dead is higher than in birds shot dead. A high level for one element did not necessarily indicate high levels for the others, and it is difficult to say how much these high levels were a cause of death, and how much they were a result of other factors that killed the guillemots. For example, some of the dead birds had rather small livers, which could increase concentrations.

Table 8-2 summarises results for PCBs and the two principal organochlorine insecticide residues. By far the most obvious feature is that the dead guillemots had very high concentrations of PCB and DDE in their livers, with much less difference from shot birds for the HEOD residues. In contrast, the two groups had rather similar concentrations in the rest of their bodies, although the shot birds tended

Table 8–1. Range of concentrations (ppm dry weight) of seven elements found in the livers of guillemots analysed at Merlewood Research Station. (Data from the Natural Environment Research Council's report.)

Source of livers	*Number of analyses*	*Lead*	*Arsenic*	*Mercury*	*Antimony*	*Zinc*	*Copper*	*Cadmium*
Birds found dead	21–22	0.8–>40	<0.1–38	<0.1–23	<0.2–410	11–600	<1–100	0.2–13
Birds shot dead	7	0.2–2.6	0.7–20	0.1–2	0.2–7	48–98	1.9–25	0.1–1.3

Table 8–2. Concentrations (ppm wet weight) of residues found in two groups of five guillemots analysed at Monks Wood Experimental Station. (Data from the Natural Environment Research Council's report.)

Tissues analysed	*Source of sample*	*Mean concentration*			*Range of concentrations*		
		PCB	*DDE*	*HEOD*	*PCB*	*DDE*	*HEOD*
Liver	Birds found dead	56	10.8	0.5	10–200	4.5–25	0.3–0.8
	Birds shot dead	0.4	0.2	0.2	0–2	0.1–0.4	trace–0.4
Rest of body	Birds found dead	3.2	0.9	0.1	1–10	0.4–2	trace–0.4
	Birds shot dead	3.4	1.5	0.5	1–7	0.6–3.1	0.2–1.0

to have larger residues. High residues in the liver do not necessarily imply that birds found dead also contained higher total amounts of residues. This difference between liver and the rest of the body could be explained, as we saw in chapter five, by supposing that the bodily changes which end in death mobilise and redistribute the body's residues, so that a relatively large part appears in the liver. The total residues in the birds' bodies supported this explanation:

	Estimated total body content (*micrograms*)					
	Mean weight			Range of weights		
	PCB	DDE	HEOD	PCB	DDE	HEOD
Birds found dead	2,700	673	62	800–8,900	314–1,535	6–232
Birds shot dead	3,500	1,484	545	800–7,200	468–3,211	155–990

Clearly these values are not over precise—the ranges are very wide and the samples of birds very small—but it was reasonable to deduce that there was no great difference between healthy and dead birds. These comparisons were based on two groups of five guillemots. The five guillemots found dead were taken from a much larger number of guillemots that had just their livers analysed. Recently J. L. F. Parslow and D. J. Jefferies have concluded, from more recent analyses of additional corpses, that these five birds were a biased sample and that in fact guillemots found dead contained on average about twice as much PCB residues in their bodies as the shot birds. This re-assessment makes PCBs a more significant factor in the guillemot wreck, and the surprisingly high percentage of adults amongst the dead birds correlates with the fact that they contained higher PCB residues than the juveniles.

To summarise, many thousands of birds died during September–November 1969. Most bodies appeared on the Ayrshire coast of Scotland at the end of September, during stormy weather, but many deaths occurred both before this when the weather was calm and later on. Levels of pollutants were not sufficiently high, compared to those in shot birds, to justify naming them as the sole cause of death. The most likely hypothesis was that, for reasons that are not at all clear, the birds were first not feeding, which caused them to mobilise their fat reserves, when levels of various pollutants increased in some tissues, and this, combined with other stresses such as the stormy weather, was sufficient to kill them.

Clearly it is difficult to draw definite conclusions from this investigation, because the data are inadequate, but there is one general point of great significance. It is reasonable to conclude that deaths resulted from a combination of factors—there was not a single cause. This is likely to be the pattern for most real-life situations.

Interactions between factors deserve a little more discussion: they may both, or all, be pollutants. Alternatively, one or more other components of the environment may also be involved. Laboratory studies have been made on the toxicity of mixtures of pairs of insecticides under controlled conditions. Sometimes such combinations are more toxic than one might expect from the toxicities of the two insecticides in isolation. One can represent this situation graphically:

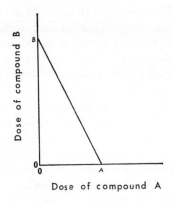

Dose of compound A

Let us suppose that a units of compound A, or b units of compound B, are, if none of the other compound is present, the LD_{50} in certain specified conditions. One might expect, if these two compounds act in the same way, that one could replace equitoxic amounts of A by B, or vice versa, and not affect the toxicity. This assumes that the effects are additive, and is represented on the graph by the straight line that joins a to b. Thus a mixture of $(a/2 + b/2)$ should also be the LD_{50} dose, as should $(\frac{1}{4}a + \frac{3}{4}b)$, and so on. This would obviously be true if compounds A and B were in fact the same compound. In practice however the toxicity of mixtures of two compounds is sometimes more than additive. Equitoxic mixtures then fall on a curve joining a and b, sweeping nearer to the origin than the straight line ab, and potentiation is said to occur. A variation on this theme is that sometimes one compound (a synergist) has virtually no effect on its own, but increases the toxicity of another. Sometimes the toxicity of a mixture is less than additive, when the compounds are antagonistic.

Synergists are of considerable practical importance with some insecticides. Pyrethrins for example are very expensive, and can be cheaper to use if synergists are included in the formulation. Because of this much work has been devoted to discovering why synergists are synergists. They all appear to act by reducing the insect's ability to metabolise the insecticide.

I made one very important qualification when discussing potentiation, that the two compounds act in the same way. Let us now suppose instead that compound A produces its primary lesion in the nervous system, whilst compound B affects the excretory system. Let us also suppose that for a specific population the LD_{40} for both compounds is half of the LD_{50}. Let us also make a third, rather improbable, assumption that if individuals from this population were arrayed in order of increasing resistance to compound A, they would also be arrayed at the same time in order of decreasing resistance to compound B. Then a dose of $(a/2+b/2)$ would kill 80% of the individuals, provided there were no interactions between the effects of A and of B. A less unlikely third assumption can be made—that arraying the individuals in order of increasing resistance to A merely leaves them in random order of resistance to B. The dose of $(a/2+b/2)$ would then kill 64% of the individuals (40% plus 40% less 40% of 40%). These examples do show that the toxicity of a mixture of compounds can be greater than simple addition might suggest, without the need to invoke interactions as the explanation. It is important to note that death is an all-or-none response. Despite the practical difficulties that may arise in deciding whether an animal is dead or alive, we may suppose, for practical purposes at least, that it is either alive or dead. Sublethal effects on the other hand can commonly be measured quantitatively on a single individual. In this situation the numerical data are sufficient by themselves to decide whether or not there is evidence of an interaction. Let us suppose we are testing the effects of $a/2$ units of compound A and $b/2$ units of compound B on the longevity of some experimental animals. In practice such situations can be very complicated, but for illustrative purposes, let us suppose we obtain the following results:

Treatment	Mean longevity (days)
Controls	100
$\dfrac{a}{2}$	80
$\dfrac{b}{2}$	70

If there were no interaction, we might expect a mean longevity, for animals dosed with $(a/2+b/2)$ units, of 50 days. A figure of less than 50 days would suggest potentiation, whereas a figure of greater than 50 days would suggest antagonism. Both are interactions.

This whole subject may at first sight seem rather academic, but there is great practical significance in such studies. For example, about 4,000 people died in London in December, 1952, from four days 'smog'—a mixture of smoke and fog. Many of the victims were elderly invalids whose chronic bronchitis was aggravated by the smog. The exact causes are uncertain, but it was probably the result of sulphur dioxide interacting with the associated mist of sulphuric acid and with smoke. None of these factors appeared sufficient, alone, to account for many, if any, of these deaths.

We have already seen that it can be quite difficult to decide whether a single pollutant has effects in the field. We have also seen that in practice there is frequently more than one pollutant present. This will not make interpretation very much more difficult unless combinations of pollutants interact in the biological effects that they produce. If they do, and we have very little knowledge on this subject, then both interpretation of data and decisions on how to control pollution will be very much more difficult to make. In practice, so far, we have tended to assume, unless there is good evidence to the contrary, that interactions are only of minor importance.

A pollutant's toxicity can also be altered by influences far more dissimilar than another pollutant, when the term 'stress' is frequently used. This has a precise meaning in physical science, where it indicates a force tending to deform a structure, and by analogy, in common parlance, it indicates some degree of hardship. It is rather more difficult to attribute a precise biological meaning to it. The best that I can suggest is, any factor which tends to displace an organism from its normal state of equilibrium. Thus low temperature can be a stress for a mammal, because it increases the amount of energy needed to maintain the body temperature. It would not necessarily be a stress for a cold-blooded fish, which would conform to the drop in temperature.

Stress is therefore a useful omnibus term, used frequently in biology to denote adverse circumstances, and there is little doubt that stresses of various sorts can increase the toxicity of pollutants. We have however little quantitative information on the subject, perhaps because it is approaching real-life situations, which are, for most experimental biologists, too complex to be worth investigating.

There is one other aspect of practical problems which is often overlooked. Normal commercial or industrial activities commonly use 'technical grade' chemicals, which contain various impurities. Laboratory experiments on pollutants commonly use very pure compounds. There is a school of thought that argues one should, in laboratory experiments on pollutants, use the normal technical grade product because the results will then approximate more closely to what might be expected to happen in the field. Clearly there is a place for this, although there are two practical difficulties. Firstly, laboratory experiments are not intended to, and rarely do, simulate field conditions. Secondly, results are difficult enough to explain when working with one known compound. The use of technical grade products means the gratuitous addition of other compounds, which, in practice, may make the experimental results useless because they cannot be interpreted and because often they cannot easily be compared with the results of other experiments. However, it is vitally important we remember that some of the impurities in technical grade products may themselves be biologically active. Their activity, and possible interactions with the principal compound, do need to be studied. I will give just two examples of such biologically active impurities.

Before we can understand our first example I must briefly recount a small part of mammalian physiology. Sexual activity in most mature female mammals occurs in distinct cycles, and the periods of heat, or oestrus, are controlled by many factors. One of the more important is a hormone, oestradiol, secreted by the ovary, which prepares the body for reproduction. Amongst other effects, the uterus enlarges. W. Levin *et al* reported, in 1968, that if 10 ppm of *op'*-DDT is injected into immature female rats then, six hours later, their uteri are 74% heavier than those of control rats. One obvious suggestion is that *op'*-DDT acts like an oestrogen, and can initiate sexual cycles. There was some corroborative evidence for this suggestion. The same response occurred in rats whose ovaries had been removed, so the pollutant could not have stimulated the ovaries to produce oestradiol. Furthermore, if oestradiol were injected two hours after an injection of *op'*-DDT, oestradiol was not taken up by the uterus. If *op'*-DDT is indeed an oestrogen, it might be expected to compete with oestradiol for binding sites in the uterus.

We have already seen that *op'*-DDT is one of the principal impurities in technical grade *pp'*-DDT. These two molecules differ only in which of two carbon atoms is linked to a chlorine atom, and yet *pp'*-DDT has very little oestrogenic activity. This is not really very surprising, because details of molecular structure are often critically important in determining hormonal activity. But it does mean that one of the byproducts of *pp'*-DDT has a potentially important effect which the pure insecticide lacks. In practice, in this instance, the problem is not likely to be significant—*op'*-DDT is rarely detected in wildlife specimens, and it appears to be metabolised quite rapidly.

Our second example was discovered by bitter experience. 2,4,5-T is a very effective herbicide, and reasonably non-toxic to mammals. Enormous quantities were used as a defoliant by the Americans during the war in Vietnam. It was alleged at this time that pregnant women in Vietnam began to produce an abnormally large proportion of deformed children. At first it was denied that this could have resulted from exposure to the herbicide, but eventually it was discovered that different batches of 2,4,5-T differ in the degree of their teratogenic effect. The active herbicide was not responsible, but the temperature during manufacture can vary, and sometimes, depending on the temperature, significant amounts of dioxins were formed. These impurities are now known to be teratogenic at very low concentrations.

We have seen in this chapter that field situations can introduce complications not usually encountered in the laboratory. It is now time to consider pollutants more fully within their context of the physical environment.

9

The Physical Environment

So far we have considered pollutants in two ways: mainly in terms of their direct biological effects, but also in terms of their chemical structure. One can also consider them in terms of the physical environment in which they occur, which can be conveniently divided into the land, water and atmosphere.

AIR POLLUTION
Air is a mixture of gases, and 'fresh air' contains on average:

Gas	% by volume of air
Nitrogen	78.03
Oxygen	20.99
Inert gases	0.95
Carbon dioxide	0.03

There is also a variable amount of water vapour.

Carbon dioxide is of particular interest. This gas does occur naturally of course, and is produced by most living organisms during respiration. It is also released in great quantities by burning fossil fuels—coal, oil and gas. Our rate of fuel consumption is, Arabs permitting, increasing all the time, and already in 1950 fuel combustion produced in one year 0.28 % of the amount of carbon dioxide already in the atmosphere. Tyndall first appreciated the significance of such additions to the environment. He suggested, in 1863, that variations in the amount of carbon dioxide in the atmosphere would alter our climate by changing the earth's surface temperature. Such a change is now considered by some to be a real possibility.

The explanation for this is quite simple. Most of the energy radiating from the earth's surface is in the infra-red part of the spectrum. Carbon dioxide absorbs such radiations. Apart from water vapour, the other gases we have listed do not. This difference is related to the fact that the molecules of these other gases consist of only one type of atom, whereas molecules of carbon dioxide and water contain two types of atom. A detailed explanation of the physical chemistry need not bother us here: the important biological fact is that the principal gaseous component of the atmosphere that is both changing in amount and capable of absorbing heat radiated from the earth is carbon dioxide.

Not all the carbon dioxide released by fuel combustion remains in the atmosphere. Other major reservoirs are the surface waters of the oceans, and living organisms. At present about 50% of this man-made carbon dioxide remains in the atmosphere, and during the decade 1958–1968 the amount of carbon dioxide in the air increased by about 0.2% per year.

It has been possible, by more subtle measurements, to deduce that the proportion of carbon dioxide had been increasing during the previous century too. The element carbon exists as several isotopes. One of these, carbon-14 (C_{14}) is radioactive, with a half-life of nearly 6,000 years. The C_{14} in the environment is continually replenished from the stratosphere, where nitrogen-14 is transmuted to C_{14} by bombardment with cosmic particles. The carbon in fossil fuels however has been locked away for a very long time and so contains very little of this isomer. Burning of this fuel will therefore dilute the C_{14} in the rest of the environment. From 1850–1950 the proportion of C_{14} in biological specimens, such as tree rings, had decreased by 1–2%—a 1–2% 'Suess effect'. This measure can no longer be used, because the tests of atomic weapons have now completely altered the amounts of C_{14} in the atmosphere.

Our main concern of course is with future prospects. If we assume a 4% annual increase in the combustion of fossil fuels, and about 50% of the consequent carbon dioxide remains in the atmosphere, then by the year 2,000 the carbon dioxide concentration in the air will have risen from its 1970 value of 320 ppm (by volume) to 379 ppm. Many assumptions must be made before we can predict what effect such a change would have on temperatures. The best estimates suggest that the temperature would rise by 0.5° C at the earth's surface, and fall by 0.5–1.0°C in the stratosphere at an altitude of 20–25 km. It is rather difficult to conclude precisely what effects such temperature changes would produce. By the year 2,000 we might be able to detect signs of climatic changes on a global scale. Speculation on this topic could go on indefinitely. I would make just two points. It is conceivable that such climatic changes could occur. If they did, they could have devastating results. It therefore behoves us to monitor the situation very carefully, although it will not be easy to detect any such climatic changes. For instance there are various natural oscillations in the earth's temperature, of which the ice ages are an extreme example. Secondly, increases of this magnitude in the concentrations of carbon dioxide in the air are unlikely to have any pronounced direct effects on individual living organisms. But the ecological effects could be very great. This potential pollutant would act not directly on individual plants or animals, but indirectly via the physical environment.

The atmosphere does not consist solely of gases—it also contains much fine particulate matter. It is a common experience that, even in the countryside, distant objects appear much clearer after rain. This is because the rain has washed down from the air many of the very small liquid droplets and solid particles, known collectively as particulates or aerosols. They are so fine that they do not readily precipitate down onto the earth's surface by force of gravity. Winds are amply sufficient to maintain them in suspension and their average half-life in the lower atmosphere is estimated to be between one and four weeks. It depends in part on the amount of snow and rainfall, which returns most of these particles to the earth's surface.

Aerosols can therefore travel considerable distances. They tend to aggregate, there are cycles of condensation and evaporation, and they are important sites of chemical reactions for gases.

Particulates derive from three sources: from land masses, for example by volcanic eruptions and dust storms; from the oceans, by evaporation of spray; and from man's activities. They are involved in the chemistry and biology of many aerial pollutants. It has been suggested that particulates will suffice to counteract the effects of the increase in carbon dioxide, because they tend to reflect incoming radiant energy from the sun, and the amounts of particulates in the atmosphere are increasing. This suggestion must be treated cautiously: particles can also absorb incoming radiant energy, and the net result is unknown. Also the increase in particulate matter may not be from pollution—some at least is probably from volcanic activity—and amounts appear to be decreasing again.

We will discuss sulphur as another important example. There are three major sources of sulphur in the air: (a) Decomposition of organic matter, which releases an estimated 100–250 million tons of sulphur each year, probably as organic sulphides, (b) Sea spray, which releases an estimated 40–50 million tons of sulphur as sulphate each year, and (c) Man's activities, which release an estimated 35–45 million tons of sulphur from the combustion of coal and oil, which contain sulphur as an impurity.

So, in the 1960s, when these data were calculated, our species contributed a minor, though important, part of the total amounts of sulphur in the world's sulphur cycle. Much of the man-made emissions occur in north-west and central Europe which, with adjacent industrialised areas, covers about 1% of the earth's surface but emits about 20% of the man-made sulphur, which is therefore, in this area, the major source. Here if anywhere one might expect pollution by sulphur, and direct damage to vegetation does occur in the Ruhr and parts of Czechoslovakia. At a lower level, differential toxicity ensures that roses grown near industrial areas are not

afflicted by the fungus that causes black spot, which is more susceptible to sulphur than is the rose. There are many other effects too,
such as corrosion of painted surfaces, stone and metal, but such costs
are normally tolerated.

Apart from this relatively local contamination though one might
hope that sulphur released by our activities might be taken into the
natural sulphur cycle without causing any damage. Recent work
suggests that this is not the case.

Sulphur can occur in many forms, and we need first to consider
what happens to the sulphur in fossil fuels when burnt. Most of it will
be oxidised and released as sulphur dioxide, although about two or
three per cent is oxidised further to sulphur trioxide, which combines
immediately with water to form sulphuric acid, a very corrosive acid.
The usual measurement for sulphur in the air is to measure the concentration of sulphur dioxide, but this is not the final stage. Water is
always present in the air, as vapour, fine droplets of water, and as a
film of moisture on small particles. Sulphur dioxide combines with
the water to form sulphurous acid, which is then oxidised to sulphuric
acid. This may be partly or completely neutralised in particulates by
acid-soluble oxides, or by ammonia taken up from the atmosphere.
All this sulphur, both acidic and neutralised, can be measured as
sulphate, but only recently have techniques been developed for
measurement of sulphuric acid (hydrogen sulphate) alone. The
distinction is important because sulphuric acid is likely to be more
harmful than is a neutral sulphate. However, some measure can be
obtained by pH, which indicates the concentration of hydrogen ions
and, in this context, can be taken as a measure of the concentration
of strong acids like sulphuric acid.

The 'beneficiaries' of industrial sulphur dioxide will of course be
downwind from the source, although this is not quite as simple as it
sounds. It must be remembered that the atmosphere has three dimen-
sions, winds can travel in different directions at different heights
above the ground, and the sulphur will not be all at one height.

It does seem that rainfall in the northern half of Europe was much
more acid in 1966 than ten years earlier in 1956:

Annual mean pH[1] value of rainfall

	1956	1959	1961	1966
Cornwall (S.W. England)	>6.0	>6.0	>6.0	>6.0
East Anglia (E. England)	5.0–4.5	5.5–5.0	5.0–4.5	4.5–4.0
Amsterdam	5.0–4.5	4.5–4.0	4.5–4.0	<4.0
Stockholm	>6.0	5.5–5.0	5.5–5.0	5.0–4.5
Lapland	>6.0	6.0–5.5	6.0–5.5	5.5–5.0

[1] The smaller the value, the greater the degree of acidity. A change of 1.0 indicates a ten-
fold change of acidity. Distilled water with dissolved carbon dioxide from the air can
attain a pH value of about 6.5.

Cornwall has retained a non-acid rainfall, whereas Lapland, which is also far from the main urban centres, now has more acidic rain than it used to. This difference is presumably related to the predominant wind directions. Air-borne particles on the south and west coasts of Sweden contain far more soot and sulphate when winds are from the south than when they are from the north, and this is consistent with the distribution of population and industry in the northern half of Europe. It has been estimated that about 9 Kg of sulphur per hectare (8 lb/acre) is deposited annually in southern Sweden, and that about half of this comes from abroad, principally central Europe and Great Britain. Does it matter?

There is evidence to suggest that the water in many Swedish lakes and rivers is becoming more acid. This assertion rests on three types of evidence: (a) Comparisons of the pH values recorded for various lakes investigated at intervals during the last forty years, (b) Comparison of the pH measured, in 1965 and 1970, at 1,000 fixed points in Scandinavia, and (c) Monthly determinations of the pH in Swedish rivers. Fifteen were selected in 1965, and the number was increased to 72 in 1969.

The general conclusion is that Swedish rivers are becoming more acid. The rate depends very much on the circumstances. In particular, for any given input of acid, the degree of acidification will depend on how hard the water is; calcium bicarbonate has a buffering effect.

It is difficult of course to explain with certainty this change in Swedish waterways. Direct discharge of acids in sewage, and less lime being used in agriculture, could both contribute, but the Swedish Government reported in 1971, to the United Nations Conference on the Human Environment, that the increasing acidity of Swedish rivers and lakes seemed to be due mainly to the deposition of sulphuric acid.

If this be true, and extensive investigations are now under way to test this, then the consequences are potentially serious. A pH of less than 5 is inimical to most animal life, and changes of pH above that value could also be expected to influence the distribution of some animals. So far though, very few observations have been made on biological changes in these affected waters. Again, as with carbon dioxide, the potential effects will be mediated via the physical environment, not by direct effects of sulphur on the aquatic organisms.

Sulphur compounds, and much carbon dioxide, come from chimneys. It has usually been considered that, given proper design and siting, dispersion of such compounds into the air is the end of the problem. To some extent this is true—gases in air are often rapidly diluted by mixing with adjacent air. This is however a local viewpoint. We have already seen for heavy metals that these problems can sometimes be properly evaluated only by taking a regional or global viewpoint.

Sulphur, and many other aerial pollutants, may eventually reach water. Pollutants in water pose rather different problems.

WATER POLLUTION

Rivers have many practical uses. In particular they both supply drinking water and act as drains to carry away our waste materials. These are conflicting activities and must therefore be controlled. In London the need for control became imperative and obvious during the early part of the last century. Amongst other developments, the last recorded salmon from the Thames was caught in 1833, and the first epidemic of cholera, which is transmitted principally by water, occurred in 1832. There has been a series of British Royal Commissions and Acts of Parliament ever since, to deal with various aspects of water pollution. The process is not yet ended. We now have a permanent Royal Commission on Environmental Pollution, and the most recent Bill, for the Protection of the Environment, had not yet reached the statute book when Parliament was dissolved in February 1974.

The biological effects of pollutants can be subsumed under a few headings, although it should be borne in mind that a pollutant may act in more than one of these ways at one time.

Firstly, some pollutants, such as washings from china clay deposits, act as inert suspensions which are deposited on the river or sea bed when the current is slow enough to allow settling. Whilst such particles are in suspension they make the river opaque and so retard or prevent plant growth. When the particles do settle they smother any algal growth, kill rooted plants and mosses, and alter the nature of the substratum.

Secondly, pollutants may be poisonous to one or more species. These poisons are derived from many industrial processes, and they can include acids and alkalis, phenols, cyanides, heavy metals and insecticides. Some, such as ammonia, are oxidised and therefore become harmless fairly rapidly, some precipitate out, and all are diluted when they mix with less polluted water. But we have to accept that many of the rivers in our industrial areas are now no more than open drains. It would be unrealistic though, even if it were economically feasible and scientifically desirable, to pipe effluents direct to the sea. We abstract so much water from our rivers that some would dry up completely except in wet weather if no effluents were returned to them.

Most of the toxicological work has been done on fish, and has usually measured the LC_{50}—that concentration which is lethal to 50 % of a group of fish, after a set time in specified conditions. Such measurements, like the LD_{50} we discussed earlier, have their place, but are of very limited use. It should be obvious by now, from previous chapters, that really we want to know the effects of these pollutants on populations in the rivers, and pollutants can affect populations in far more subtle ways than simple acute toxicity. It must be agreed that ecological studies on rivers are difficult, but even at the physiological level we have amazingly little knowledge. Given the practical need for studies on the effects of mixtures of pollutants in rivers, physiological studies on interactions could be very useful and should not be too difficult.

Thirdly, some pollutants combine with oxygen in the water, and in extreme cases may completely deoxygenate the water. Different species require different minimal oxygen concentrations, but few can survive without any. The amount of oxygen actually present is the balance between many processes. In brief, oxygen gets into water by photosynthesis and by solution from the surface. It is lost by respiration, sometimes by heating, and by chemical reaction. Inorganic pollutants such as sulphides and sulphites react immediately with any oxygen in the water, but many oxidisable organic pollutants use up oxygen more slowly—the oxidation depends on bacteria, whose activity will depend on numbers, temperature, presence of other nutrients, and so on. Organic pollutants can breakdown to some extent even if no oxygen is present. This process of putrefaction can lessen, although not eliminate, the oxygen debt, because unoxidised volatile components such as methane (marsh gas), ammonia and hydrogen sulphide are released into the atmosphere. Here again, as we saw with aerial pollutants, organisms are affected indirectly. One can hardly call lack of oxygen a poison, but it will certainly keep out many plants and animals.

It is obviously important that we can assess the ability of sewage to deoxygenate water. It is impracticable to do this by measuring the concentrations of specific deoxygenating compounds, in part because there can be so many of them, especially organic molecules, and also because this alone would not tell us the rate at which oxygen will be used up, but only the total amount. The British Royal Commission on Sewage Disposal therefore recommended, in 1912, the five-day Biochemical Oxygen Demand test (BOD). We must examine this test in some detail before we can appreciate both its uses and its limitations. The sample of effluent or river water is diluted with sufficient well oxygenated water to ensure that about half the oxygen will still be present at the end of the test. The sample is then stored, in a stoppered bottle, at 20°C, in the dark to prevent any photosynthesis, for five days, when the amount of oxygen (mg) used by 1 litre of the sample is measured. If 3 mg of oxygen were used per litre, the result would be expressed as a BOD of 3 ppm.

To give some idea of scale, sewage from one human being requires about 100 g of oxygen per day, which represents the total amount of oxygen that can be dissolved in about 2,000 gallons of water at normal temperatures. A major preoccupation in sewage works is to minimise the BOD of the effluent, so as to minimise river pollution.

Many artefacts are possible with this test, which may give a misleading impression of safety. For example the effluent may contain compounds that inhibit the bacteria, and so reduce the rate of oxidation. The appropriate bacteria may be absent, or they may lack other necessary nutrients. It is possible to overcome these and other difficulties, but the test is most reliable when comparing similar effluents.

One might hope, knowing the BOD of an effluent, to predict the amount of oxygen in a river below the outfall. This is often feasible, but the calculation can be very complicated, because so many factors affect the rates of both oxidation of the pollutant and oxygenation of the water. Oil for instance, even as a thin surface film, reduces the rate of oxygenation from the air.

The Royal Commission classified reaches of rivers by various criteria—amount of suspended matter, smell, abundance and types of organisms—into five categories. They found that the BOD test (determined at 65°F) was the best single chemical index of the degree of pollution in a waterway, and the mean values from a series of rivers correlated very well with the categories of the reaches sampled:

Category	Number of waterways sampled	BOD(ppm) Mean	BOD(ppm) Range
Very clean	7	1	0.0– 2.6
Clean	24	2	0.1– 5.0
Fairly clean	28	3	0.5– 7.0
Doubtful	8	5	1.6–12.7
Bad	5	10	2.3–26.4

BOD is still an important criterion of river quality, but it is important to note that there was a considerable range of values for samples from sites in the same category. Some of this variation was inevitable, because chemical values for rivers vary from time to time, but it is uncertain how complete an explanation this is.

Fourthly, some pollutants are nutrient salts that enhance plant growth. This process of eutrophication can occur naturally, and it is

I

most easily studied in lakes. If a lake's drainage area contains only rocks and infertile soils then its water will contain only small amounts of nitrate, phosphate and potassium, the major plant nutrients, and the biological productivity will be small. Such a lake is said to be oligotrophic. At the other extreme, a eutrophic lake contains large amounts of the major nutrients, and productivity is high. In time oligotrophic lakes can sometimes naturally become eutrophic. The total biomass increases, and the species change because the balance of advantage between species changes as the environment changes.

Two aspects of eutrophication have caused particular complaint. The amount of phyto-plankton (small free-living plants) increases, and sometimes algal blooms occur, which then die and deoxygenate the water. Blooms are unlikely to occur in rivers, in the UK at least, because the algae will be continually removed downstream, although problems may develop later if the water is then stored in lakes or reservoirs. Such blooms can destroy the amenity value of a lake, some of the algae release toxins that can kill fish and livestock, and the algae make the water less suitable for drinking and for many industrial purposes. Another major complaint is that eutrophic lakes tend to contain less desirable fish than do oligotrophic ones. For instance, roach may replace trout.

Such changes have occurred in some lakes and rivers by man's activities, although we do not fully understand why and when eutrophication causes algal blooms. Sometimes they do not occur even though conditions appear suitable. Presumably there are many interacting factors, and some of these interactions are as yet unknown. However, the consensus of opinion is coming to be that phosphorus (as phosphate), derived largely from sewage, is a key factor.

It is a very nice question whether the release of additional phosphate into waterways is pollution. It may just accelerate the process of eutrophication that sometimes occurs in due course by natural processes. There is little doubt though that the accelerated change is undesirable.

The important question, as always, is what effects pollution produces on the biology of a waterway. We have already seen that our knowledge of biological effects is rather scanty, and a survey made in 1970 of river pollution in England and Wales emphasised how unable we are as yet to predict the biological consequences of river pollution. 16,532 miles of waterway were assessed for water quality by both chemical and biological criteria. The chemical criteria, which included the occurrence of polluting discharges, BOD, dissolved oxygen, turbidity, absence of fish and frequency of complaints, provided four grades:

(1) Unpolluted or recovered from pollution
(2) Of doubtful quality, many needing improvement
(3) Of poor quality, improvement needed as a matter of some urgency
(4) Grossly polluted

These waterways were also put into four grades after a biological assessment, based on the numbers and species diversity of both fish and invertebrates:

(a) Widely diverse invertebrate fauna, and good fisheries
(b) Varied invertebrate fauna, and good fisheries, although salmon and grayling absent even if ecological factors favourable
(c) Restricted invertebrate fauna, moderate to poor fisheries
(d) No invertebrate fauna, or a few resistant species only, and no fish life

Pollution is by definition a biological phenomenon, so one might hope that these two sets of criteria would give similar conclusions. Unfortunately the correspondence was less than expected:

Chemical grade	Miles of river	Miles of river that had corresponding biological grade	% agreement between criteria
1	12,827	10,241	80
2	2,195	1,228	56
3	748	427	57
4	762	572	75

More work needs to be and is being done on this topic, because river quality is normally assessed by chemical criteria.

LAND

Man is a terrestrial species, and our major impact, over many centuries or even millenia, has been on the land. Unlike the other two components of the physical environment, land is not fluid, and so it is that the most obvious effects have been physical transformations. Agriculture, urban development and mining have all altered the land surface. There is probably nowhere in Great Britain where the flora is truly wild, in the sense that there is no part of the flora that has been unaffected by man's activities. A lot of our flora is semi-natural, in the sense that it has come of its own accord, but that is not quite the same thing.

We have to accept as a fact that we are now the dominant species on our planet and that we can, either inadvertently or deliberately, damage very rapidly the world's biological productivity and diversity.

I wish briefly to discuss just one aspect of the creation of new terrestrial environments. The extraction of large quantities of minerals can create one or both of two problems: what to do about the hole, and what to do with the waste material. The simple answer, to fill the hole with the waste material, is not always possible. It would not be very easy to put slag from metal mines back into the pits, and sometimes the slag is produced so far from the pit that it is uneconomic to return it.

Waste materials obliterate the original surface soil, and one approach has been to attempt to create new soils out of the waste material that will support plant growth on the heaps. Obstacles can be severe. There may be physical problems of poor water retention, unsuitable texture for plant growth and lack of stability. There may be chemical problems of lack of nutrients, presence of toxins, or unsuitable degree of acidity or alkalinity.

For example, a large coal-burning power station may use several million tons of coal in a year, and a fifth of this may be left as ash. These large piles of ash could perhaps be landscaped into acceptable contours, a layer of top soil added, and vegetation established. However, top soil is both expensive and difficult to get. So experiments are going on into the use of 'ameliorants' such as peat or river silt, with artificial fertilisers, which are mixed thoroughly into the surface layer of the pulverised fuel ash to produce a synthetic soil. It is early days yet to decide how successful such schemes will be.

This approach, if successful, will serve to epitomise our dominating influence on our environment.

10

Pollution in Perspective

I have not attempted to mention all pollutants—catalogues have their uses for practitioners, but rarely make for stimulating reading. I have tried rather to develop a point of view, which I have illustrated by some specific examples. It seems appropriate to end by considering some of the wider implications.

A recurring theme has been the discovery of new pollutants by accident, in two senses of that word. One is bound to ask therefore how many pollutants still await discovery. Recent estimates suggest that we are producing about 100 million tons of organic chemicals per year, of which about one fifth may enter the environment. The range of compounds is considerable, and it must be wellnigh impossible to investigate each compound, and all the possible interactions with other potential pollutants.

There appear to be two complementary ways in which we can try to avoid serious trouble from all the possible, but unknown, hazards. For substances, metabolites and break-down products that are persistent and for which there are adequate analytical methods, it is possible to analyse samples at regular intervals. These samples may come from both the physical and living environments, and the area sampled can range from a small site near an emission source to the whole globe. Worthwhile results can only be obtained if there is meticulous attention to detail at the planning stage, and resources can very rapidly become the limiting factor. Chemical analyses are expensive and time-consuming, and budgets for large programmes very rapidly become enormous. The alternative approach is to measure the size of specific populations of plants or animals. Again this could be very expensive, at least in man-hours, but it has often been done, especially for birds, by large numbers of enthusiastic and knowledgeable amateurs. Of course many changes other than pollution can affect populations, but if there is a sudden change in numbers then it may be worth making a more intensive study of the reasons why. Many of our pollution problems so far have first been detected by their biological effects in the field.

These activities are commonly referred to as monitoring. The term monitor used to indicate periodic surveys made to ensure that specific residues did not exceed set limits in particular samples. It now usually has the looser meaning of periodic surveys made to detect any changes, either in residues of pollutants or in numbers of organisms.

Monitoring can only be regarded though as a first line of defence. Ideally we would never have unexpected incidents. They occur because we lack sufficient knowledge. I would argue that the proper remedy is for more research—previous chapters have, I hope, indicated some of the problems that need to be tackled. This argument is not universally accepted—some criticism runs along the lines that technology has produced most of the current unpleasant aspects of life, such as pollution, and that the only sensible thing to do is to revert to a much simpler way of life. Many of us do have our own private version of some idyllic pastoral existence, but I am not convinced that, at present, more than a small minority would wish to return, even if it were possible, to a less technological way of life. Even then, we would still retain some of our current problems, although to a lesser degree. Rather we have to accept, and act on, the fact that we can no longer leave things to chance—our overall impact on the environment is too great.

Incomplete experimental evidence, or results from monitoring, sometimes make it prudent to control some form of pollution before there is complete proof of damage. The peregrine falcon is a good example. Critics of such proposed controls often make much play of the incomplete nature of the evidence. This is sometimes a little surprising when it comes from commercial interests. Businesses are invariably run on inadequate information and by extrapolation—managers can only try to make the best judgement possible from the available information. The same applies to pollution. If we waited for proof before acting, we would sometimes be too late. Adequate control of pollution sometimes requires international agreements. If a conflict of interests occurs at this level, resolution can be very difficult.

So far we have considered the unknown problems. Many are known, and require little or no research. We cannot assume that known problems will be solved automatically. It is perhaps inevitable that the economic system makes solutions difficult. One simple, and perhaps simplified, example may make this clear. Commercial firms can only remain viable so long as they make a profit. Costs are of two sorts—internal and external. External costs are those which are not borne by the firm, but by the rest of the community. There might be a new oil burning plant to be installed. It is technically possible to remove much of the sulphur from the waste gases and prevent its emission into the atmosphere. Unless there are legal constraints, the decision will rest, at least in part, on the relative costs of sulphur recovered from the flue gases and sulphur bought on the world market. Any costs to others, if the sulphur is not removed, will not enter into the calculation. Given the system, this is unavoidable, and conflicts of interest are inevitable. And the problem cannot always be settled within the confines of one country alone. The country that has strict controls on pollution increases the costs of its products. Firms from other countries that have less strict controls will have a competitive advantage. At this stage the argument becomes one of economics, suggests the need for administrative controls, and is rather beyond my competence to discuss. But the simple fact remains that if we want to reduce pollution we must be prepared to pay for it. More pollution control means less of some other desirable thing. In current terms, we have to make decisions about the quality of life.

Control of pollution means that decisions have to be made, and controls imposed. It is therefore essential that as much relevant information as possible be available. Archaic ideas still persist, sometimes overtly, that it is undesirable for information to be freely available. For example, pollutants in effluent wastes poured by factories into rivers are still a confidential matter between the individual firm and the river authority. I have no reason to suppose that the inspectorate is less than perfect, in an imperfect world, in achieving the proper balance in the control of waste discharges. However, this being so, there is no reason why the figures should not be available to all who wish to see them. It is sometimes argued that such figures would reveal vital information about a firm's products to its competitors, but this sounds more like an excuse than a rational argument. It is true that publicity sometimes entails a lot of ill-based scaremongering, but this hardly justifies secrecy, which can encourage even more improbable rumours. I started this book by quoting, from a White Paper, the need for a well-informed and active public opinion. I concur, and would conclude that adequate control of pollution, like freedom, requires eternal vigilance.

Bibliography

JOURNAL ABBREVIATIONS

Adv. ecol. Res.	*Advances in Ecological Research*
Ann. appl. Biol.	*Annals of Applied Biology*
Arch. environ. Health	*Archives of Environmental Health*
Br. J. ind. Med.	*British Journal of Industrial Medicine*
Calif. Fish Game	*California Fish and Game*
Can. Ent.	*Canadian Entomologist*
Chem. Ind. Lond.	*Chemistry and Industry*
Entomol. Gaz.	*Entomologist's Gazette*
Environ. Polln.	*Environmental Pollution*
Environ. Qual. Saf.	*Environmental Quality and Safety*
Fed. Am. Soc. exper. Biol.	*Federation of American Societies for Experimental Biology*
Geochim. Cosmochim. Acta	*Geochimica et Cosmochimica Acta*
J. appl. Ecol.	*Journal of Applied Ecology*
J. Biol. Chem.	*The Journal of Biological Chemistry*
J. econ. Ent.	*Journal of Economic Entomology*
J. Fish Res. Bd. Can.	*Journal of the Fisheries Research Board of Canada*
J. Wildl. Manage.	*The Journal of Wildlife Management*
Pestic. Monit. J.	*Pesticides Monitoring Journal*
Proc. R. Soc. Edin.	*Proceedings of the Royal Society of Edinburgh*
Proc. R. Soc. Lond.	*Proceedings of the Royal Society of London*
Sci. Total Environ.	*The Science of the Total Environment*
Toxic. appl. Pharmac.	*Toxicology and Applied Pharmacology*
World Neurol.	*World Neurology*

The references are of two sorts. Some are mentioned specifically in the text. Others deal more fully, and or more technically, with certain aspects.

Chapter 1.
Office of the Secretary of State for Local Government and Regional Planning. *The Protection of the Environment: the Fight against Pollution* (London, H.M.S.O. 1970, Cmnd. 4373).

Chapter 2.
Hartley, G. S. & West, T. F. *Chemicals for Pest Control* (Pergamon Press, 1969).
Harvey, G. R., Steinhauer, W. G. & Teal, J. M. Polychlorobiphenyls in North Atlantic Ocean Water, *Science, N.Y.* **180** (1973), 643.
Jager, K. W., Roberts, D. V. & Wilson, A. Neuromuscular Function in Pesticide Workers, *Br. J. ind. Med.* **27** (1970), 273.
Jensen, S., Renberg, L. & Olsson, M. PCB Contamination from Boat Bottom Paint and Levels of PCB in Plankton outside a Polluted Area, *Nature, Lond.* **240** (1972), 358.

Maugh, T. H. DDT: an Unrecognised Source of Polychlorinated Biphenyls, *Science, N.Y.* **180** (1973), 578.
Mellanby, K. *Pesticides and Pollution* (London, Collins, 2nd ed. 1970).
O'Brien, R. D. *Insecticides: action and metabolism* (New York, Academic Press, 1967).
Prestt, I., Jefferies, D. J. & Moore, N. W. Polychlorinated Biphenyls in Wild Birds in Britain and their Avian Toxicity, *Environ. Polln.* **1** (1970), 3.
Risebrough, R. W., Huggett, R. J., Griffin, J. J. & Goldberg, E. D. Pesticides: Transatlantic Movements in the North East Trades, *Science, N.Y.* **159** (1968), 1233.
Woodwell, G. M., Craig, P. P. & Johnson, H. A. DDT in the Biosphere: Where Does it Go? *Science, N.Y.* **174** (1971), 1101.

Chapter 3.
Lockie, J. D., Ratcliffe, D. A. & Balharry, R. Breeding Success and Organo-chlorine Residues in Golden Eagles in West Scotland, *J. appl. Ecol.* **6** (1969), 381.
Ratcliffe, D. A. Changes Attributable to Pesticides in Egg Breakage Frequency and Eggshell Thickness in some British birds, *J. appl. Ecol.* **7** (1970), 67.
Ratcliffe, D. A. The Peregrine Population of Great Britain in 1971, *Bird Study*, **19** (1972), 117.

Chapter 4.
Cooke, A. S. Shell Thinning in Avian Eggs by Environmental Pollutants, *Environ. Polln.* **4** (1973), 85.
Erben, H. K. & Krampitz, G. Eischalen DDT-verseuchter Vögel: Ultrastruktur und organische Substanz, *Abhandlungen der mathematisch-naturwissenschaftlichen Klasse, Akademie der Wissenschaften und der Literatur, Mainz* (1971), 31.
Hazeltine, W. Disagreements on why Brown Pelican Eggs are Thin, *Nature, Lond.* **239** (1972), 410.
Switzer, B. C., Wolfe, F. H. & Lewin, V. Eggshell Thinning and DDE, *Nature, Lond.* **240** (1972), 162.
Wiemeyer, S. N. & Porter, R. D. DDE Thins Eggshells of Captive American Kestrels, *Nature, Lond.* **227** (1970), 737.

Chapter 5.
Borg, K., Wanntorp, H., Erne, K. & Hanko, E. Alkyl mercury Poisoning in Terrestrial Swedish Wildlife, *Viltrevy*, **6** (1969), 301.
Chadwick, G. G. & Brocksen, R. W. Accumulation of Dieldrin by Fish and Selected Fish-food Organisms, *J. Wildl. Manage.* **33** (1969), 693.
Cooke, A. S. Selective Predation by Newts on Frog Tadpoles treated with DDT, *Nature, Lond.* **229** (1971), 275.
Coulson, J. C., Deans, I. R., Potts, G. R., Robinson, J. & Crabtree, A. N. Changes in Organochlorine Contamination of the Marine Environment of Eastern Britain Monitored by Shag Eggs, *Nature, Lond.* **236** (1972), 454.

Dimond, J. B., Belyea, G. Y., Kadunce, R. E., Getchell, A. S. & Blease, J. A. DDT Residues in Robins and Earthworms Associated with Contaminated Forest Soils. *Can. Ent.* **102** (1970), 1122.

Hayes, W. J. Pharmacology and toxicology of DDT. In *DDT: The Insecticide Dichlorodiphenyltrichloroethane and its Significance*. Vol. II, edited by Simmons, S. W. (Basel, Birkhaüser Verlag, 1959), 11.

Hayes, W. J., Dale, W. E. & Pirkle, C. I. Evidence of Safety of Long-term, High, Oral Doses of DDT for Man, *Arch. environ. Health*, **22** (1971), 119.

Holden, A. V. International Cooperative Study of Organochlorine Pesticide Residues in Terrestrial and Aquatic Wildlife, 1967/1968, *Pestic. Monit. J.* **4** (1970), 117.

Hunt, E. G. & Bischoff, A. I. Inimical Effects on Wildlife of Periodic DDD Applications to Clear Lake, *Calif. Fish Game*, **46** (1960), 91.

Hunter, C. G., Robinson, J. & Roberts, M. Pharmacodynamics of Dieldrin (HEOD). Ingestion by human subjects for 18 to 24 months, and post-exposure for eight months, *Arch. environ. Health*, **18** (1969), 12.

Jefferies, D. J. & Davis, B. N. K. Dynamics of Dieldrin in Soil, Earthworms, and Song Thrushes, *J. Wildl. Manage.* **32** (1968), 441.

Meeks, R. L. The accumulation of ^{36}Cl ring-labelled DDT in a freshwater marsh, *J. Wildl. Manage.* **32** (1968), 376.

Moore, N. W. & Walker, C. H. Organic Chlorine Insecticide Residues in Wild Birds, *Nature, Lond.* **201** (1964), 1072.

Moriarty, F. The Effects of Pesticides on Wildlife: exposure and residues, *Sci. Total Environ.* **1** (1972), 267.

Moriarty, F. Residues in Animals during Chronic Exposure to Dieldrin, *Environ. Qual. Saf.* **3** (1974), 104.

Moriarty, F. Exposure and residues. In *Organochlorine Insecticides: Persistent Organic Pollutants*, edited by Moriarty, F. (London, Academic Press, 1975), 29.

Reinert, R. E. Accumulation of Dieldrin in an Alga (*Scenedesmus obliquus*), *Daphnia magna*, and the Guppy (*Poecilia reticulata*), *J. Fish. Res. Bd. Can.* **29** (1972), 1413.

Chapter 6.

Antonovics, J., Bradshaw, A. D. & Turner, R. G. Heavy Metal Tolerance in Plants, *Adv. ecol. Res.* **7** (1971), 1.

Askew, R. R., Cook, L. M. & Bishop, J. A. Atmospheric Pollution and Melanic Moths in Manchester and its environs, *J. appl. Ecol.* **8** (1971), 247.

Busvine, J. R. Mechanism of Resistance to Insecticide in Houseflies, *Nature, Lond.* **168** (1951), 193.

Dempster, J. P. The Control of *Pieris rapae* with DDT. II. Survival of the young stages of *Pieris* after spraying, *J. appl. Ecol.* **5** (1968), 451.

Dempster, J. P. Some Observations on a Population of the Small Copper Butterfly *Lycaena phlaeas* (Linnaeus) (Lep., Lycaenidae), *Entomol. Gaz.* **22** (1971), 199.

Dempster, J. P. Effects of organochlorine insecticides on animal populations. In *Organochlorine Insecticides: Persistent Organic Pollutants*, edited by
Moriarty, F. (London, Academic Press, 1975), 231.

Moriarty, F The Toxicity and Sublethal Effects of p,p'-DDT and Dieldrin
to *Aglais urticae* (L.) (Lepidoptera: Nymphalidae) and *Chorthippus brunneus*
(Thunberg) (Saltatoria: Acrididae), *Ann. appl. Biol.* **62** (1968), 371.

Soliman, S. A. & Cutkomp, L. K. A Comparison of Chemoreceptor and
Whole-fly Responses to DDT and Parathion, *J. econ. Ent.* **56** (1963), 492.

Weigedal, J. E. & Harper, A. E. Metabolic Adaptations in Higher
Animals. IX. Effect of high protein intake on amino nitrogen catabolism
in vivo, *J. biol. Chem.* **239** (1964), 1156.

Chapter 7.

Ackefors, H. Mercury Pollution in Sweden with Special Reference to
Conditions in the Water Habitat, *Proc. R. Soc. Lond.* B, **177** (1971), 365.

Hammond, P. B. The Relationship between Inhibition of δ-Aminolevulinic
Acid Dehydratase by Lead and Lead Mobilization by Ethylenediamine-
tetraacetate (EDTA), *Toxic. appl. Pharmac.* **26** (1973), 466.

Kurland, L. T., Faro, S. N. & Siedler, H. Minamata Disease, *World
Neurol.* **1** (1960), 370.

Murozumi, M., Chow, T. J. & Patterson, C. Chemical Concentrations of
Pollutant Lead Aerosols, Terrestrial Dusts and Sea Salts in Greenland and
Antarctic Snow Strata. *Geochim. Cosmochim. Acta.* **33** (1969), 1247.

National Academy of Sciences, *Biologic Effects of Atmospheric Pollutants.
Lead. Airborne Lead in Perspective* (Washington, D.C. 1972).

Parslow, J. L. F., Jefferies, D. J. & French, M. C. Ingested Pollutants in
Puffins and their Eggs, *Bird Study*, **19** (1972), 18.

Preston, A., Woodhead, D. S., Mitchell, N. T. & Pentreath, R. J. The
Impact of Artificial Radioactivity on the Oceans and on Oceanography,
Proc. R. Soc. Edin. B, **72** (1971/72), 411.

Rissanen, K. & Miettinen, J. K. 2. Use of Mercury Compounds in
Agriculture and its Implications. In 'Mercury Contamination in Man and
his Environment', Technical Report Series no. 137, International Atomic
Energy Agency, Vienna, 1972.

Chapter 8.

Hewlett, P. S. Synergism and Potentiation in Insecticides, *Chem. Ind.
Lond.* no. 22 (1968), 701.

Holdgate, M. W. (editor). The Sea Bird Wreck in the Irish Sea Autumn
1969, *The Natural Environment Research Council, Publication Series C no.* **4**
(1971).

Levin, W., Welch, R. M. & Conney, A. H. Estrogenic Action of DDT and
its Analogs, *Federation Proceedings. Fed. Am. Soc. exper. Biol.* **27** (1968), 649.

Parslow, J. L. F. & Jefferies, D. J. Relationship between organochlorine
residues in livers and whole bodies of guillemots, *Environ. Polln.* **5** (1973), 87.

Chapter 9.

Hynes, H. B. N. *The Biology of Polluted Waters* (Liverpool University Press, 1960).

Report of the Study of Critical Environmental Problems, *Man's Impact on the Global Environment* (M.I.T. 1970).

Sweden. Royal Ministry for Foreign Affairs & Royal Ministry of Agriculture. *Air Pollution across National Boundaries: the Impact on the Environment of Sulfur in Air and Precipitation; Sweden's Case Study for the United Nations Conference on the Human Environment*, (Stockholm, 1972).

Index